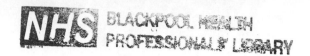

The Dental Nurses' Guide to Infection Control and Decontamination

The Dental Nurses' Guide to Infection Control and Decontamination

by
Kathryn Porter

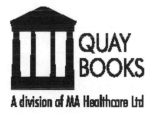

QUAY
BOOKS

A division of MA Healthcare Ltd

Quay Books Division, MA Healthcare Ltd, St Jude's Church, Dulwich Road, London
SE24 0PB

British Library Cataloguing-in-Publication Data
A catalogue record is available for this book

© MA Healthcare Limited 2008
ISBN-10: 1 85642 360 3   ISBN-13: 978 1 85642 360 1

Printed by Ashford Colour Press, Gosport, Hants PO13 OFW

Contents

Note
While the authors and publishers have made every effort, as far as is possible, to confirm the information in this book complies with the latest standards of practice and legislation, the authors and the publishers cannot take responsibility from any instances arising as a result of errors. Healthcare practice and knowledge are constantly changing and developing.
Practitioners are encouraged to seek help where they are not competent to carry out a procedure.

Foreword

The prevention of infection is fundamental to all aspects of today's healthcare system, ensuring a safe environment for both the patient and healthcare worker alike. The practice of infection prevention in dentistry has never been as high on the political agenda as the public responds to their concern of healthcare associated infections. Blood-borne viruses continue to influence healthcare practice and procedures in an effort to reduce the incidence of transmission to and from healthcare workers (HCWs). The emergence of the degenerative brain diseases caused by prions (often manifested as Creutzeldt-Jacob disease with its resistance to decontamination procedures), particularly demand attention from dental nurses (and others responsible for decontamination) who are usually responsible for such processes.

Clinical techniques have improved and progressed, but new procedures are not without risk to both the patient or the healthcare worker, none more so than the dentist and dental nurse as it can be argued that by its very nature every dental procedure is invasive and potentially will put all at risk from coming into contact with body fluids.

The design of a dental surgery is fundamental to modern dentistry and thus effect infection control procedures to become routine and 'design out' risks of cross contamination.

The risk of transmission from infected patient-to-HCWs is greater than HCW-to-patient, but specialists in dentistry can unwittingly put their patients at risk of exposure via contaminated instruments, so it is pleasing to find a chapter on the care and maintenance of instruments within this book.

This book is an excellent resource with up-to-date references for today's dental nurse, practising in both primary care and acute dentistry such as dental teaching hospitals. This book is a compendium of knowledge for a dental nurse working in a variety of practice settings. I have no hesitation in recommending this book to dental nurses and as a reference manual for infection control nurses.

Kathleen Hughes
Infection Control Nurse Specialist and Decontamination Lead,
Birmingham East and North PCT

Acknowledgements

I would like to thank the following for their considerable assistance and support with the production of this book.

Fiona Blair, Consultant in Restorative Dentistry (Periodontology), Honorary Senior Lecturer, Infection Control Lead, Birmingham Dental Hospital, for validating and advising on the technical content.

Angela Dann, Senga David, Elizabeth Mills, Tutor Dental Nurses, Birmingham Dental Hospital, for proof reading the chapters and giving advice on the content.

Janice Dukes, Curriculum Co-ordinator, Oral Health and Tutor, Matthew Boulton College, Birmingham, for advice from a general practice standpoint.

Introduction

This book is aimed at giving an insight into the complex and ever changing subject of infection control and decontamination for dental nurses working in any branch of dentistry. The very nature of infection means that new variants and strains are emerging constantly, so it is important that dental nurses keep up-to-date with the changes and amend their practices accordingly.

This book is aimed at being a practical guide, giving background information and theory and practical guidance on how to implement this knowledge. It is by no means exhaustive. Current research being undertaken will also throw up new ideas and prove or disprove present theory and practice as will the challenges presented by new instruments and dental procedures. During the preparation of this book, updated guidance was published by the Chief Dental Officer, on the disposal of endodontic files which will have a significant impact on general dental practitioners.

The information given is correct at the time of going to print, but should not be taken as an unchanging fact. It is the responsibility of all dental practitioners to keep up-to-date with changes, and this now includes dental nurses with the advent of State Registration and its requirement for Continued Professional Development (CPD).

Infection control must be the first consideration when any changes are planned in dental surgeries. The wellbeing of the patient must always be the overriding consideration. There must never be any chance of any infection being passed from one patient to another, or to staff. It is essential that efficient infection control and decontamination underpins all practices and procedures undertaken and becomes second nature for all members of the dental team.

The British Dental Association (BDA) leaflet A12 *Infection Control in Dentistry* (BDA, 2003) must always be the source of reference and the information contained in it used as the minimum requirements for each and every dental practice. Practices should have infection control and decontamination policies in place and these should form part of the induction of new staff into the practice. These policies should be regularly reviewed to take account of changes in official advice. Hospitals and Personal Dental Services will have their own infection control policies which should be followed at all times. These again should be regularly reviewed in the light of new research. It has been suggested that yearly infection control training should become part of the mandatory training schedule and should certainly be part of CPD for all the dental team.

It is important to recognise that non-compliance with policies is not an option as there are legal requirements for everyone under various acts of Parliament that govern different aspects of infection control and decontamination.

Decontamination of equipment, instruments and the disposal of waste are integral responsibilities of the dental nurses' job, but this does not preclude them from being supervised and controlled by the dentist in a general practice, or by line managers within the hospital or private dental service. Decontamination practices will change with the advent of new research and in response to new infections. It is imperative that this subject remains part of DPD for all dental team members and it should form part of regular review during team meetings.

Please note that the legislation quoted is legislation mainly relating to England and Wales. Some legislation will cover all countries of the UK, but there are specific regulations for Scotland, Northern Ireland and in some cases, Wales. The best advice is, if living outside England, check what the relevant regulations are for your area. Advice can be found from the various web sites named in the resources section of this book.

Glossary

Aerosol: Dispersion of solid or liquid particles in a gas.

Antisepsis: The destruction or inhibition of micro-organisms on living tissues having the effect of limiting or preventing the harmful results of infection.

Antiseptic: A chemical agent used in antisepsis.

Bowie-Dick Test: Test designed to indicate that a steriliser is capable of removing air and non-condensable gases from a load.

Carrier: A person (host) who harbours a micro-organism (agent) in the absence of discernible clinical disease. Carriers may shed organisms into environment intermittently or continuously and therefore act as a potential source of infection.

Cleaning: The process that physically removes soiling including large numbers of micro-organisms and the organic material on which they thrive.

Clinically-acquired infection: Infection acquired during clinical/therapeutic care; not present or incubating at the start of the care/treatment.

Colonisation: The presence of micro-organisms at a body site(s) without the presence of symptoms or clinical signs of illness or infection. Colonisation may be a form of carriage and is a potential method of transmission.

Commensal: A micro-organism resident in or on a body site without causing clinical infection.

Communicable period: The time in the natural history of an infection during which transmission may take place.

Contamination: The presence of micro-organisms on a surface or in a fluid or material.

Decontamination: The combination of processes, including cleaning, disinfection and/or sterilisation, used to render a reusable item safe for further use.

Disinfectant: A chemical agent which, under defined conditions, is capable of disinfection.

Disinfection: The reduction of the number of viable micro-organisms on a product to a level previously specified as appropriate for its intended further use.

Epidemic: An unusual, higher than expected level of infection or disease by a common agent in a defined population in a given period.

Flora: Micro-organisms resident in an environmental or body site.

Hospital-acquired–Infection (nosocomial infection): Infection acquired during hospitalisation; not present or incubation at the time of admission to hospital.

Immunity: The resistance of a host to a specific infectious agent.

Immuno-compromised: A state of reduced resistance to infection that results from malignant disease, drugs, radiation illness or congenital defect.

Incidence: The number of new cases of a disease (or event) occurring in a specified time.

Incubation Period: The time interval between initial exposure to the infectious agent and the appearance of the first sign or symptoms of the disease in a susceptible host.

Infection: The damaging of body tissue by micro-organisms or by poisonous substances released by the micro-organisms.

Isolation: The physical separation of an infected or colonised host from the remainder of the 'at risk' population in an attempt to prevent transmission of the specific agent to other individuals and patients.

Medical Device: An instrument, apparatus, appliance, material or other article, whether used alone or in combination, together with any software necessary for its proper application, which is used for human beings for the purpose of healthcare treatment, diagnosis, prevention or monitoring. It also includes accessories necessary for the correct functioning of the medical device.

Micro-organisms: A microscopic entity capable of replication. It includes bacteria, viruses and the microscopic forms of algae, fungi and protozoa.

Operating Cycle: The set of stages of the sterilisation or disinfection process carried out in sequence and regulated by the automatic controller. It is synonymous with the terms sterilisation cycle for sterilisers and disinfection cycle for disinfectors.

Pathogen: A micro-organisms capable of producing disease.

Potable Water: Water of a suitable quality for drinking, cooking or food production.

Reusable Device: A medical device which can be reprocessed for repeated episodes of use.

Reservoir: Any animate or inanimate focus in the environment in which an infectious agent may survive and multiply and which may act as a potential source of infection.

Seroconversion: The development of antibodies not previously present resulting from a primary infection.

Sharps: Sharps are items that could cause cuts or puncture wounds. They include needles, hypodermic needles, scalpel and other blades, knives, infusion sets and broken glass.

Single Use: A medical device that is intended to be used on an individual patient during a single procedure and then discarded. It is not intended to be reprocessed and used on another patient.

Source: Place where micro-organisms are growing or have grown.

Sterile: Free from all living micro-organisms.

Sterilisation: A process which renders an item sterile.

Sterilising Agent: An agent or combination of agents which, under defined conditions, leads to sterilisation.

Surveillance: A systematic collection, analysis and interpretation of data on specific events (infections) and disease, followed by dissemination of that information to those who can improve the outcome.

Susceptible: A person presumably not possessing sufficient resistance (or immunity) against a pathogenic agent who contacts infection when exposed to the agent.

Transmission: The method by which any potentially infecting agent is spread to another host.

Ultrasonic Cleaners: A machine which uses ultrasound energy to effect mechanical removal of soiling from the surface of the product.

Virulence: The intrinsic capabilities of a micro-organism to infect a host (person) and produce disease.

Washer / Disinfector: A machine intended to clean and disinfect medical devices and other articles used in the context of medical, dental, pharmaceutical and veterinary practice.

WEEE: Waste Electrical and Electronic Equipment (in relation to European commission Directive 2002/96/EC).

WM2: Technical document produced by the Environment agency, Scottish Environment Protection Agency, and the Environment and Heritage service to provide guidance on the assessment and classification of Hazardous Waste, based on the Hazardous Waste Directive definition of hazardous waste.

Resources

Within Dentistry

British Association of Dental Nurses: www.badn.org.uk
British Dental Association: www.bda-dentistry.org.uk
British Dental Health Foundation: www.dentalhealth.org.uk
British Dental Hygienists Association: www.bdha.org.uk
British Dental Practice Managers Association: www.bdpma.org.uk
British Orthodontic Society: www.bos.org.uk
Clinical Dental Technicians Association: www.cdta.org.uk
Dental Nursing: www.dental-nursing.co.uk
General Dental Council: www.gdc-uk.org
Orthodontic Technicians Association: www.orthota.co.uk
World Dental Federation: www.fdiworldental.org

Non Dental-Specific

Centres for Disease Control and Prevention (USA): www.cdc.gov
Department of Health: www.doh.gov.uk
Health and Safety Executive: www.hse.gov.uk
NHS Scotland: www.show.scot.nhs.uk
Northern Ireland Health Department: www.dhsspsni.gov.uk
Welsh Health Information: www.wales.gov.uk/subihealth/index/htm

There are thousands of other sites on the Internet, both in the UK and worldwide, accessible by searching with key words, such as 'infection', 'steriliser', 'dentistry', etc. Additionally, each Primary Care Trust have their own websites and often post their own policies on it, which are accessible to the public.

CHAPTER 1

What is Infection?

Infection is the invasion and multiplication of micro-organisms within the tissue, which then results in their destruction. This is often seen as a chain of events (*Figure 1*). Each link in the chain must be present, and in the sequential order shown, for an infection to occur. Understanding the different links in the chain provides healthcare professionals with methods to protect vulnerable people and thereby prevent the spread of infection.

If any one of the links in the chain is broken or eliminated, then the infection can be prevented or the spread of infection reduced.

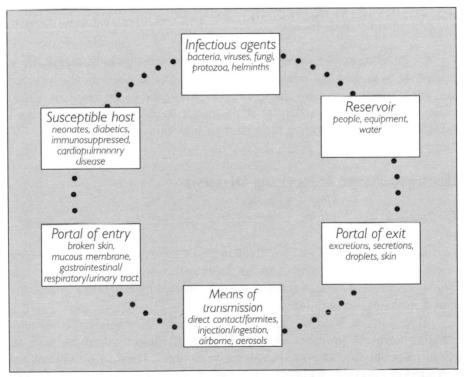

Figure 1. The chain of infection. If any of these links are broken infection could be prevented or reduced.

What is Infection Control?

Infection control is the prevention of the spread of infections within a healthcare setting, and it is an essential part of the infrastructure of healthcare.

Infection control concerns itself not only with the investigation and management of the spread of an infection in an area, but also with the prevention of infections arising. It is because of this dual responsibilities that it is usually known as Infection Control and Prevention.

Infection control consists of three main areas:

- **Hand hygiene**: it is well documented that ineffective or non-existent hand hygiene is a major factor in the spread of infections
- **Cleaning, disinfection and sterilisation**: the effective cleaning, disinfection and sterilisation of equipment is the only sure way to prevent infections passing from one person to another. Although this system does not destroy prions, the agents responsible for CJD
- **Personal protective equipment**: this is essential to protect the healthcare worker from being infected by anything spread from a patient and *vice versa*.

All these areas will be explained fully in the following chapters. It is important to understand what infectious diseases are, how they are spread and what causes them. This makes the prevention and control of their spread easier to arrange. It also underpins all the measures taken to prevent infections occurring and for controlling the spread of infections already present.

Background to Infectious Disease

Definition

An infectious disease is one which damages or injures the person as a result of the presence and activity of one or more pathogenic, microbial agents. It can be transmitted through contact with an infected individual by inhalation, inoculation, ingestion or infestation.

Infections can be contracted by a member of the dental team through inhaling aerosols produced during the use of airotors, sonic scalers or cavitrons, or by the aerosols splashing into the eyes. They are also at risk for inoculation (needlestick) injuries from sharp needles or burs, matrix bands, or other sharp tools.

A contagious disease is an infectious disease that is capable of being transmitted from one person to another. It can be transmitted by direct contact with an individual, contact with body fluids or with objects that the infected individual has contaminated. The prevention of the spread of these diseases is the reason for decontamination and sterilisation of equipment and surfaces.

Pathogens

A pathogen is a biological agent that causes disease or illness to its host. It can also be known as an infectious agent. This term is most often used to describe an agent which disrupts the normal physiology of a plant or animal.

Relatively few micro-organisms cause disease in a healthy individual. Infective disease results from the interaction between pathogenic micro-organisms and the body's defences. The severity of the resulting disease is dependant on the ability of the pathogen to damage the host and the ability of the host's defences to resist the pathogen.

Pathogens are classified as either primary or opportunistic.

Primary Pathogens

These cause disease as a result of their presence or activity within a normal healthy host. The severity of the disease is in part a consequence of their need to reproduce and spread. They will cause a more severe disease in a host which has a more depressed resistance than is normal.

Opportunistic Pathogens

These cause infectious diseases in a host with depressed resistance. These pathogens are often in contact with the host or could be acquired from another host, or from the environment. It requires the host to have impaired defences which could be caused by genetic defects, by exposure to certain drugs, such as chemotherapy drugs or by immunosuppressive therapy, or in other vulnerable groups such as those with a low nutritional status.

The Body's Defences

Micro-organisms have six routes of entry into the body:

- Skin and mucous membranes
- Inhalation
- Ingestion
- Injection
- Implantation
- Transmission through the placenta *in utero*.

The human body has in-built defences to repel the attack of pathogenic micro-organisms. These in-built defences can be divided into two groups:

- Non-specific defence mechanisms (NSDM)
- Specific defence mechanisms (SDM).

Non-Specific Defence Mechanisms

Skin
Skin is the first line of defence. The skin contains an inherent waterproofing protein, keratin, which provides a barrier to the entrance of micro-organisms. Also, the skin has a natural regular shedding of the upper surface layer, the dermis, allowing for a large number of micro-organisms to be removed from the skin.

Chemical Factors and Body Fluids
Chemical factors also have an important role to play in the resistance of microbial invasion. Sebum is secreted from the sebaceous glands which contains unsaturated fatty acids which in turn inhibit the growth of bacteria and fungi. Skin is naturally acidic caused by the secretion of these fatty acids and lactic acid, which deters the growth of micro-organisms.

Sweat glands produce perspiration, which flushes microbes from the skin surface. Sweat also contains enzymes which are capable, under certain conditions, of breaking down the cell walls of certain bacteria. These enzymes are also present in nasal secretions, tears and saliva and tissue fluids. The shedding of sweat, saliva and tears helps prevent the colonisation of some micro-organisms.

The one-way flow of urine also acts as a cleansing factor, similarly vaginal secretions in women help to wash microbes out of the body.

Mucous Membranes
Mucous membranes line all the body cavities that are open to the outside environment, i.e. the gastrointestinal tract, respiratory tract, genito-urinary tract and the reproductive tract. These membranes also secrete mucus which is very viscous (sticky), which not only stops the cavities from drying out, but also traps micro-organisms and inhibits their growth.

The mucous membrane in each different tract has structures which are specific to that area and help to prevent microbes entering their particular system. For example, hairs in the nose trap microbes, dust and pollutants. Cilia in the respiratory tract pass unwanted particles, which have been trapped in the mucous, up to the throat. The epiglottis prevents particles entering the trachea.

Gastric juices
Micro-organisms entering the stomach are destroyed by the gastric juices which are a mixture of hydrochloric acid, enzymes, and mucus. Gastric juices have a high acidity and ensure that the stomach remains sterile.

The body has other ways of eliminating foreign bodies, including microbes through coughing, sneezing, vomiting and diarrhoea.

Coughing
This is the body's natural reaction to foreign bodies being swallowed into the trachea instead of the oesophagus and, in times of infectious attack, of dispelling micro-organisms from the lungs.

Sneezing
This is the body's natural reaction to foreign bodies, including pathogens invading the upper respiratory tract, especially the nose.

Vomiting
This is the body's natural response to infectious materials in the stomach by removing the offensive material.

Diarrhoea
This is the body's way of ridding the body of infectious or pathogenic micro-organisms in the lower digestive system.

Phagocytosis

Blood also has in-built defence mechanisms to combat micro-organisms should they breach the initial defences and enter the body. These are principally made up of various types of white blood cells. The process by which white blood cells (also known as T-cells) defend the body against attack is known as phagocytosis.

When microbes infect the body the white blood cells migrate to the affected area where they pass through the wall of the blood vessel to attack the invader. Phagocytosis is made up of four stages:

- *Chemotaxis*: chemical attraction of white cells to micro-organism and damaged cells
- *Adherence*: the attachment of a blood cell to micro-organism
- *Ingestion*: the blood cells completely encloses the micro-organism
- *Digestion*: the blood cell digests the micro-organism by using enzymes, bacterial substances and hydrogen peroxide.

Phagocytosis at the site of an infection results in the symptoms of heat, redness, swelling, pain and loss of function. This is known as an inflammatory response and is the body's attempt to dispose of toxins and foreign materials. The fever produced decreases microbial activity by decreasing the optimum conditions for growth and speeds up the body's natural defence reactions.

Interferon

The body also produces antimicrobial substances known as interferons. These chemicals are released into the blood and have different responsibilities in the fight against infection and are essential for the formation of T-cells

Interferons in general have several effects in common. They are antiviral and possess antioncogenic properties, macrophage and natural killer lymphocyte activation, and enhancement of major histocompatibility complex glycoprotein classes I and II, and thus presentation of foreign (microbial) peptides to T-cells. In a majority of cases, the production of interferons is induced in response to microbes such as viruses and bacteria, as well as mitogens and other cytokines, for example interleukin 1, interleukin 2, interleukin-12, tumor necrosis factor and colony-stimulating factor, that are synthesised in the response to the appearance of various antigens in the body. Their metabolism and excretion take place mainly in the liver and kidneys. They rarely pass the placenta but they can cross the blood-brain barrier.

Inflammation

The substances responsible for inflammatory response are histamine, kinins, prostaglandins, leucotrienes and complement. The presence of these substances results in vasodilation and the increased permeability, which enables antibodies, phagocytes and clot forming chemicals to enter the area of attack.

In the absence of inflammation, wounds and infections would never heal and progressive destruction of the tissue would compromise the survival of the organism.

Fibrin

Fibrin is a protein involved in the clotting of blood. It is a fibrillar protein that is polymerised to form a 'mesh' that forms a hemostatic plug or clot (in conjunction with platelets) over a wound site.

Fibrin is formed which is carried to the site of injury where it traps the pathogens, forming a clot, sealing the wound to prevent any more micro-organisms entering.

Specific Defence Mechanisms

Specific defence is known as immunity. This is the production of a specific antibody for each pathogen. Foreign organisms, or antigens, stimulate the immune response to produce antibodies which are produced by lymphocytes. Antigens are chemicals produced by foreign bodies, usually micro-organisms, which stimulate the host lymphocytes to produce antibodies to neutralise them.

Antibodies are chemicals produced by the body to counteract the actions of infectious pathogens. Antibodies (also called immunoglobulins) enhance phagocytosis, neutralise toxins and trigger the complement system to protect the body from bacterial and viral attack. Antibodies are proteins that are found in blood or other bodily fluids of vertebrates, and are used by the immune system to identify and neutralise foreign objects, such as bacteria and viruses. Antibodies are produced by a kind of white blood cell called a B-cell. There are several different types of antibodies, and each help direct the appropriate immune response for each different type of foreign object they encounter. Although the general structure of all antibodies is very similar, a small region at the tip of the protein is extremely variable, allowing millions of antibodies with slightly different tip structures to exist. This region is known as the hypervariable region. Each of these variants can bind to a different antigen. This huge diversity of antibodies allows the immune system to recognise an equally wide diversity of antigens.

Recognition of an antigen by an antibody tags it for attack by other parts of the immune system, for example T-cells. Antibodies can also neutralise targets directly by, for example, binding to a part of a pathogen that it needs to cause an infection.

The body uses two responses to combat foreign bodies: cell-mediated immunity and humoral immunity.

Cell mediated immunity
This involves T-cells latching onto the foreign material and destroying it. The presence of antigens in turn stimulates the production of T-cells.

Humoral immunity
This involves the production of antibodies which circulate in the blood and which invade and attack pathogens. Antibodies are made by B-cells.

T-cells and B-cells are both different types of white blood cells. Both are produced in lymph tissue and are common in lymph nodes and, to a lesser extent, in the spleen, gastro-intestinal tract and bone marrow.

During the processing of antigens, interleukin and interferon are secreted which stimulate more T-cell growth. When sensitised by coming into contact with antigens, T-cells increase in size and divide, giving rise to clones known as Memory T-cells, Helper T-cells, Killer T-cells and Suppressor T-cells. Each has a different function in the fight against the infectious pathogen.

Specific Considerations

HIV
The number of T-cells present in the blood is used as a test to monitor human immunodeficiency virus (HIV) sufferers. It tests the number of CD4 T-cells present in the blood. If the CD4 count falls it is a sign of the progression of the HIV infection. If the CD4 count falls below 200 cells/mm^3, the HIV infection is officially diagnosed to have become acquired immune deficiency syndrome (AIDS). This is often coupled with the emergence of certain opportunistic infections.

Transplants
Unfortunately, the body has the same immune response to the 'invasion' of a transplanted foreign body, i.e. heart, kidney or liver. This can lead to tissue rejection which is inherent in the normal body defence response against invasion. Hence the need for anti-rejection drugs and a possible reduction in the body's normal response to infection. These are important considerations when treating patients who have had transplants.

Agents of Infection

There are five main types of infectious agents:

- Viruses
- Bacteria
- Fungi
- Protozoa and arthropods
- Prions.

Viruses

Viruses are the smallest pathogenic micro-organisms which have to be studied using scanning or transmission electron microscopes. Viruses cannot reproduce themselves outside the body; they can only replicate themselves by infecting a host cell and using the machinery and metabolism of the host cell to produce copies of themselves. Viruses infect a wide variety of organisms, animals, plants, fungi and also bacteria. However they can live outside the body for varying lengths of time.

Viruses are made up of genetic material contained in a protective protein coat called a capsid. They are not made up of cells. There are four main virus types:

- Helical viruses (example: Tobacco Mosaic virus)
- Icosahedral viruses (example: Hepatitis B virus)
- Enveloped viruses (example: Influenza or HIV virus)
- Complex viruses (example: bacteria-infecting viruses).

Viruses cause diseases in humans, such as the common cold, chickenpox, cold sores, HIV/AIDS, influenza and rabies. The ability of viruses to cause disease is described in terms of their 'virulence'. Viruses can be transmitted by direct contact, via body fluids or through a vector (for example certain mosquitoes).

Viruses are difficult to eliminate from a host because they depend on the host cells to reproduce and they reside in them, and therefore killing the virus can also kill the host cell. Antibiotics have no effect on viruses and there are few effective antiviral drugs available at present. The best way to prevent viral diseases is by vaccination which produces immunity. Drugs can be taken to alleviate the symptoms.

Viruses can only be destroyed from external surfaces by sterilisation.

Bacteria

Bacteria are unicellular micro-organisms presenting in many shapes, including spheres (Cocci), rods (Bacilli) and spirals (Spirilla or Spirochetes). They are found in all environments. They are both beneficial in some forms and detrimental in others.

Beneficial bacteria are present throughout our body, for example in the intestinal and genital tract. There are approximately 10 times as many bacteria cells as human cells in a human body. There are large numbers present on the skin and in the digestive tract. The body's own immune systems render the majority of these bacteria either harmless or beneficial, but some do cause infectious diseases. Detrimental types of bacteria (pathogenic bacteria) cause infections such as cholera, syphilis, leprosy and tuberculosis. The most common fatal bacterial diseases are those which cause respiratory diseases.

Bacteria show a large diversity of cell morphologies and arrangements and often join together in characteristic patterns. For example, *Streptococcus* forms chains; *Staphylococcus* forms 'bunches of grapes' clusters; *Actinobacteria* form elongated filaments.

Bacteria can attach themselves to surfaces, forming dense groups called biofilms or microbial mats. Biofilms have significance in chronic bacterial infections and infections on implanted medical devices because they are much harder to kill than individual bacteria. These biofilms and microbial mats are of importance in decontamination of dental water lines, as will be described in a later chapter, and it is for this reason that it is advisable to disinfect the skin prior to giving injections or inserting indwelling catheters (which will be discussed in later chapters).

Bacteria are known as Gram positive and Gram negative. This relates to the structure of the bacteria cell wall and its ability to take up a stain (Gram positive) or not (Gram negative), when examined under the microscope. The differences in structure between Gram positive and Gram negative bacteria can influence antibiotic susceptibility. For example, vancomycin will only kill Gram positive bacteria and is totally ineffective against Gram negative bacteria.

Bacteria are killed by antibiotics which are either bacteriocidal (kill bacteria) or bacteriostatic (inhibit growth and reproduction). One of the main problems with diseases caused by bacteria is that the bacteria can develop resistance to the antibiotics being used to destroy it. This is exacerbated when bacteria are exposed inappropriately to the antibiotics (when antibiotics are prescribed for viral infections and when used extensively in farm animals).

Bacteria reproduce by cell division and under optimal conditions can grow and divide rapidly. Populations can double in as few as 10 minutes. They can move about using flagella, by gliding, twitching or by changing their buoyancy. Different species have differing numbers and arrangements of flagella on their surface. Some bacteria produce endospores which can lie dormant for millions of years and resist destruction by UV light, gamma radiation, detergents, disinfectants, heat, pressure and extreme dryness, for example *Clostridium tetani* whose spores lie in the soil and cause tetanus infections if they contaminate wounds.

Surface bacteria are killed by sterilisation and some can be killed by disinfection using, for example, bleach.

Fungi

Fungal infections are also called mycoses and are classified according to the tissue levels initially colonised:

- Superficial: limited to outer layers of skin and hair
- Cutaneous: extends deeper into the epidermis as well as invasive hair and nail diseases. They can produce an immune response from the host
- Subcutaneous: chronic infections and initiated by piercing trauma to the skin allowing fungi to enter. These diseases may need surgical debridement to treat
- Systemic mycoses: are due to primary pathogens, they originate in the lungs, primarily and can spread to other organs

- Systemic mycoses: are due to opportunistic pathogens which affect people with immune deficiencies who would not normally be affected.

Common fungal infections include athlete's foot and ringworm, both of which are readily passed from one person to another. In the case of ringworm it is contagious before it shows positive symptoms. Athlete's foot is caused by microfungi, the spores of which are carried in the air.

Candida, a common opportunistic systemic mycosis, is caused by a yeast.

Fungi are made up of threadlike cells called hypha (plural hyphae). These cells group together to form mycelium which may produce a fruiting body as a means of reproduction. The most common and easily recognised are mushrooms in all their various forms.

Protozoa and Arthropods

Protozoa are single cell animals. Beneficial protozoa have important roles in the decomposition of food materials and control of bacterial populations. Pathogenic protozoa produce diseases such as malaria.

Arthropods are also known as parasites. There are three main groups of parasites:

- Endoparasites: they live inside the host body (for example gut worms)
- Ectoparasites: they live on the outside of the host (for example fleas)
- Epiparasites: they live on other parasites and are mainly found in the insect population.

Endoparasites can enter the host through broken skin, but mainly enter via the consumption of raw foods which have been contaminated by the parasite's eggs; they produce huge numbers of eggs which are excreted and then inadvertently ingested by others when food is not properly washed. They are prevalent in areas of poor sanitation when the water supplies are also contaminated so that even if food is washed it is not parasite-free.

Ectoparasites are passed from host to recipient by close contact with either the individual or with contaminated items. For example, fleas can jump from host to recipient, lice can be transmitted by direct contact or through contaminated clothing, hair brushes, etc. They are sometimes known as 'social parasites'. They can cause infectious reactions in the host body and bites can cause infections to arise.

Most parasites cannot live for long away from the host as they feed by sucking blood from the host. They are killed by sterilisation and disinfection.

Prions

The term 'prion' stands for protinaceous infectious particle and describes an infectious agent made only of protein. They are responsible for causing diseases known as transmissible spongiform encephalopathies, the most notorious of which for humans is Creutzfeldt-Jakob disease (CJD) and its variant (vCJD). These diseases affect the brain and neural tissue and are untreatable and fatal.

The proteins that prions are made up of are found throughout the bodies of both infected and healthy people. The prion protein found in infectious material has a different structure and is resistant to the enzymes within the body which normally break down proteins to amino acids. Prions resist digestion in the gut and remain intact. It is thought that they pass into lymph tissue and from there to the brain and neural tissues.

Prion infections can be inherited and a mutant gene has been identified in these cases, in many different forms. CJD and vCJD are, primarily, transmitted to humans from the meat or brains of infected animals. They resist destruction by high temperatures, so will resist destruction during the cooking process of infected meat.

There is a great deal of research being undertaken to fully understand the mechanism of prion infection and reproduction. A specific committee has been set up to review the research being carried out. This committee is known as the Spongiform Encephalopathy Advisory Committee (SEAC). Its latest position statement was published in June 2007. One of its conclusions was that preliminary research findings suggest that the potential risk of transmission of vCJD via dental procedures may be greater than previously anticipated (SEAC, 2007).

Prions are not killed by sterilisation. However, the main risk is of cross contamination is from instruments used on specific tissue types. These include lymphoid tissue, eye and brain tissue. There is also a remote risk from pulpal tissue in teeth. Instruments not used in these specific instances can be sterilised in the normal way as there is little risk of prions being present.

Transmission of Infections / Infectious Diseases

Infection control and decontamination is all about avoiding infections and infectious diseases being passed from one patient to another or to the dental professional. To understand the need for various types of infection control and policies, it is important to understand how infections and infectious diseases are transmitted from one host to another recipient. Understanding how a disease is transmitted helps to understand the biology of the infectious agent and helps in combating the disease it causes. Transmission takes five main routes:

- Inhalation
- Ingestion
- Inoculation
- Via body fluids
- Vectors.

Inhalation

Infectious agents causing respiratory diseases and meningitis are commonly spread by inhalation of aerosol droplets spread by sneezing, coughing, talking, singing. They can also be spread by inhaling aerosol droplets formed during dental treatment using airotors and sonic scalers or cavitrons.

Ingestion

Gastrointestinal infections are often acquired by digesting contaminated food or water. This would include food prepared by people who have an infection and who do not perform effective hand hygiene or food not washed effectively before consumption. It will also include food washed in contaminated water.

Inoculation

Pathogenic micro-organisms can enter the body through damaged skin, via cuts and abrasions, or by inoculation by dirty needles or other sharp instruments contaminated by body fluids, or by bites from insects.

Via Body Fluids

This group contains four main routes:

- **Blood**. Serious infections carried in the blood include hepatitis in all its variants, and HIV. They can be transmitted by contamination through an uncovered wound

13

or abrasion or by inoculation such as a sharps injury. There is also, in dentistry, the danger of transmission through splashing into the eyes or inhalation of aerosols produced during clinical procedures.

- **Saliva**. It is known that hepatitis infections can be active in saliva, putting the dental professionals at risk of infection by inhalation of aerosols, splashing or inoculation injuries.

- **Sexually transmitted diseases**. These are infections passed directly from one person to another as a direct result of sexual activity.

- **Infections transmitted from mother to infant via the placenta or breast milk**. These are infections present in the mother and passed through the placenta during pregnancy or via breast milk during breast feeding. These can include HIV.

Vectors

Vectors for carrying and transmitting pathogens can be either mechanical or biological.

Mechanical Vectors
These pick up an infectious agent from outside the host and transmit it in a passive manner. For example, a housefly lands on cow dung thus contaminating its legs with bacteria. The fly then lands on unprotected food, which it contaminates with its legs. The food is then eaten, possibly infecting the person eating it. The bacteria never enters the housefly.

Biological Vectors
These carry a pathogen within their body and actively deliver it to a new host, usually through a bite. They are responsible for serious blood-borne illnesses, such as malaria. Examples of biological vectors are usually arthropods such as mosquitoes, ticks, fleas and lice.

Blood and saliva are also vectors of infection if inoculated via needle stick or sharps injury or by inhalation or splashing.

The treatment of vector borne diseases is to interrupt the life cycle of the pathogen by killing the vector.

Methods of Preventing Infection

The micro-organisms which cause infectious and contagious diseases are everywhere in the environment. We live with them all day and every day; it is only when they breach our body's defences that they become dangerous to us. A prime example of this is the *Staphylococcus aureus* bacteria which live on our skin without causing us any harm, but if it enters the body through an open wound or if we become weakened by illness, it has the potential to start an infection.

How do we prevent infection from a potential pathogen which the patient we are treating may be carrying, and conversely what can we do to prevent us from infecting our patients?

This question is almost as complex as the variety of pathogens previously described. In basic terms, nothing must pass from patient-to-patient, patient-to-staff, staff-to-patient, or staff-to-staff.

It is essential that all patients have a full medical history taken at their initial visit, which is checked at each subsequent visit. All clinically involved staff should have a hepatitis B inoculation and regular blood tests to test their immunity, although there is a school of thought that believes that once initial immunity is confirmed this does not need to be checked regularly. Staff should also be aware of their immunity status for other infections such as tuberculosis, measles, mumps and rubella.

It is well and widely documented that not all patients know they are carrying an infection (and there are some patients who may not admit it). For example, hepatitis in its many forms can be carried by a person who has never been ill with the disease or had any idea that they are infected. It is for this reason, and to be fair and equitable to all patients, that Universal Precautions specifically for the prevention of infection transmission were first defined. This title has since been amended to Standard Precautions.

Universal Precautions

Universal Precautions were probably first outlined by the Centres for Disease Control and Prevention (CDC) based in Atlanta, USA (CDC, 1987). These were initially issued as recommendations for prevention of HIV transmission. The document gives in-depth advice on precautions which should be taken to protect healthcare professionals, as well as other patients, from the transmission of pathogens and has sections specifically concerned with different aspects of healthcare, including dentistry. The document emphasises that precautions should be consistently used for *all* patients. It goes on to outline in detail how healthcare workers can protect themselves and their patients from blood- and body fluid-borne infections. Precautions listed are:

- Use of personal protective equipment, including gloves, masks, goggles or face shields, gowns or disposable aprons
- Effective and timely hand washing
- Prevention of needlestick injuries
- Use of shields if giving mouth-to-mouth resuscitation
- Covering any skin wounds.

The document outlines additional precautions to be taken in dentistry and states that:

> *'Blood, saliva and gingival fluid from ALL patients should be considered infective.'*

CDC, 1987

The document advises the use of a rubber dam, high speed aspiration and the correct positioning of the patient to reduce the generation of aerosols. It goes on to describe the need for sterilisation of handpieces and the need for the flushing of water lines. It advises the thorough and careful disinfection of items to be sent to laboratories and the covering of surfaces that cannot be sterilised.

A full description of this guidance is given in later chapters.

Standard Precautions

The name Universal Precautions was later changed to Standard Precautions because it was felt that 'universal' implies perfection and, although comprehensive, these precautions cannot give perfect protection.

More recently the British Dental Association (BDA) brought Standard Precautions up-to-date and made them relevant to current dental practice (BDA, 2003). Standard Precautions have been updated to include:

- The use of personal protective equipment
- Effective hand washing
- Safe disposal of sharps
- Safe disposal of clinical waste
- Effective hard surface decontamination
- Effective decontamination and sterilisation of contaminated items
- Use of zoning techniques to prevent contamination of unsterilisable items
- Safe storage of sterilised items.

All of these components will be fully explained in subsequent chapters.

This guidance from the BDA must be the basis of infection control procedures for all dental practices. Even though these precautions are to be used for all patients, there are some additional precautions which should be taken for known infectious patients. Additional precautions (which will be described fully in a later chapter) should be taken for patients with known:

- Prion contaminations (example: CJD or vCJD)
- Airborne transmissible diseases (example: tuberculosis)
- Droplet transmissible diseases (example: mumps, influenza)
- Transmission by direct or indirect contact with dried skin (example: colonisation by MRSA or contaminated surfaces).

Standard Precautions should be also followed by all staff that come into contact with infected materials or areas.

It is also a fact that many infectious diseases are more infectious before external signs are apparent, such as chicken pox and measles, so strictly applied Standard Precautions will greatly reduce any chance of infection.

Single Use Items

There are a growing number of instruments and items of personal protective equipment which are designated by the manufacturers as 'single use'. The list of instruments falling into this category has just been lengthened following a letter from the Chief Dental Officer which categorically states that all endodontic instruments must be single use to reduce the risk of transmitting CJD or vCJD (Department of Health [DH], 2007). The list will no doubt continue to grow as these items once used on a patient are disposed of and therefore there can be no chance of any contamination being carried from one person to another.

The Medicines and Healthcare Products Regulatory Agency (MHRA) has published advice on single use items and I strongly suggest that you read it (MHRA, 2006).

Single use items are clearly marked with an internationally and legally recognised symbol (see *Figure 2* overleaf). Whenever this symbol appears on the packaging of any item, it must be obeyed. This symbol means that the item must only be used on one patient. If an item is used more than once, then any product liability which could be claimed against the manufacturer in case of fault is nullified and passes to the user, who would be liable under law for any consequences.

Figure 2. Items marked with this symbol mean that they are destined for 'single use' only and must not be used on more than one patient.

Legal Obligations and Infection Control

There is, at present, no case law specifically related to infection control and non-compliance with practices and policies. However, there are a number of Acts that have aspects which relate to infection control prevention.

The Health Act 2006 (DH, 2006) is the primary legislation which sets out the basic rules that all NHS organisations, provider organisations and private practices must comply with when dealing with prevention and control of infections. Even though not specifically mentioned, all non-NHS establishments will be expected to comply with the provisions of the Act and the Healthcare Commission Standards. It relates to the provision of healthcare directly by NHS organisations and is presented under three headings:

- NHS organisations have a general duty of care ensuring that appropriate management systems are in place to protect patients, staff and others from healthcare acquired infections (HCAI)
- Relates to clinical procedures, placing a duty of care on NHS organisations to adhere to care policies applicable to the prevention and control of HCAI
- NHS organisations have a duty to ensure, as far as possible, that healthcare workers are free of and protected from exposure to communicable infections during the course of their work. They must also have the necessary education to prevent and control HCAI.

The following is a very brief summary of the most relevant legislation, and it is strongly advised that you read the full documents. All of these can be found at the Department of Health website (www.dh.gov.uk).

The Health and Safety at Work Act 1974

This Act sets out a framework that places a duty of care upon employers and employees to promote high standards in the workplace as well as protecting the public from workplace dangers.

Section 2 makes a legal requirement, as far as is reasonably practical, for employers to create a safe working environment.

Section 7 also places an onus of responsibility and co-operation upon the individual (DH, 1974).

Management of Health and Safety at Work Regulations 1999

These regulations take into law the requirements of three EEC Directives. The Framework Directive 89/39/EEC, Council Directive 91/383/EEC and Council Directive 94/33/EC. These directives address issues of training, risk assessment and development of health and safety policies. Two further regulations were added in 1999. Regulation 4 requires employers to put in place preventative and protective measures. Regulation 21 means that the employer can be prosecuted for the actions of an employee (DH, 1999).

Control of Substances Hazardous to Health 1988 (COSHH)

These are regulations designed to prevent workplace diseases caused by substances used in the workplace. It lays down regulations to ensure that any substances which can cause harm to staff or patients are assessed. This assessment has to be written down and kept, updated and be accessible should an accident happen. The assessment will note any maximum exposure limits and any first aid and follow up treatment that is necessary should the substance be splashed, ingested or inhaled by a member of staff or a patient (DH, 1988).

Environmental Protection Act 1990

This Act sets the legal guidelines for the safe disposal of waste in all its forms and has particular meaning for healthcare establishments with its rules for the disposal of contaminated waste, sharps and clinical waste. It also sets standards and rules for the disposal of substances such as mercury and waste amalgam (DH, 1990).

There are also many national initiatives which are aimed at reducing HCAI and improving infection control. They include:

NHS Decontamination Project 1999

This programme sets out the requirements for decontamination services as a result of Medical Devices Directive 93/42/EEC. This Directive sets stringent requirements for the decontamination of all reusable medical devices and came to effect on 1st April 2007. From this date all healthcare facilities should be complying with its recommendations (NHS, 1999).

Winning Ways Guidelines
This report by the Department of Health gives clear directions to local NHS organisations on the actions necessary to reduce the high levels of HCAIs (DH, 2003).

A Matrons Charter
This document sets out broad principles for delivering cleaner hospitals (NHS, 2004).

Towards Cleaner Hospitals and Lower Rates of Infection
This document sets out a programme and strategy to improve hospital cleanliness to tackle HCAIs (DH, 2004).

Cleanyourhands Campaign
This campaign from the National Patient Safety Agency (NPSA) was rolled out in the acute sector and aims to improve hand hygiene amongst healthcare workers, patients and visitors and was extended to the primary care sector in 2007. It addresses the fact that HCAIs are spreads by inefficient hand hygiene (NPSA, 2004).

Saving Lives Campaign
This was a programme introduced to reduce HCAI such as MRSA. Although initially aimed at acute hospitals, it has benefits for all healthcare settings (DH and NHS Modernisation Agency, 2005).

All of these initiatives and guidelines further reinforce the need for compliance with local and national policies. Although primarily aimed at cutting HCAI rates in hospitals, many of the recommendations, policies and procedures outlined are pertinent to dental practices.

The *NHS Decontamination Project*, which came into force on the 1st April 2007 (NHS, 1999), sets out minimum standards for the decontamination and sterilisation of contaminated medical devices, which must be complied with by all healthcare establishments and has huge implications for dental practices.

With the registration of dental nurses, you will be governed by the standards and codes of conduct as set by the General Dental Council (GDC), our registering body. The GDC has the power to discipline, and even strike off, professionals who do not comply with the agreed standards. Putting patients at risk by following poor infection control and decontamination regimes could initiate such disciplinary action. It is important that you bear in mind at all times that preventing cross-infection is not an option, but a legal requirement.

References

BDA (2003) *Infection Control in Dentistry: Advice Sheet A12*. British Dental Association, London

Centres for Disease Control (1987) *Recommendations for the Prevention of HIV Transmission in Healthcare Settings. CDC,* Atlanta, USA

DH (2007) *Important Advice for Dentists on Re-use of Endodontic Instruments and variant Creutzfeld-Jacob Disease (vCJD): Letter from Barry Cockroft, Chief Dental officer for England*. DH, London

DH (2006) *The Health Act 2006 – Code of Practice for the Prevention and Control of Healthcare Associated Infections*. HMSO, London

DH and NHS Modernisation Agency (2005) *Saving Lives: A Delivery Programme to Reduce Healthcare Associated Infection including MRSA*. DH and NHS Modernisation Agency, London

DH (2004) *Towards Cleaner Hospitals and Lower Rates of Infection. A Summary of Action*. HMSO, London

DH (2003) *Winning Ways: Working Together to Reduce Healthcare Associated Infections in England: Report from the Chief Medical Officer* HMSO, London

DH (1999) *Management of Health and Safety at Work Regulations 1999*. HMSO, London

DH (1999) *Environmental Protection Act 1999*. HMSO, London

DH (1988) *Control of Substances Hazardous to Health (COSHH) Regulations 1988*. HMSO, London

DH (1974) *Health and Safety at Work Act 1974*. HMSO, London

Medicines and Healthcare Products Regulatory Agency (2006) Single-use Medical Devices, Advice for Healthcare Professionals. MHPR, London

National Patient Safety Agency (2004) *Cleanyourhands Campaign*. NPSA, London

NHS (2004) *A Matrons Charter: An Action Plan for Cleaner Hospitals*. HMSO, London

NHS (1999) *NHS Decontamination Project 1999*. NHS Estates, London

SEAC (2007) *Position Statement*. Spongiform Encephalopathy Advisory Committee, London

CHECKLIST 1

What is Infection?

- Chain of Infection

What is Infection Control?

Infectious disease: a disease which damages or injures the person as a result of the presence and or activity of one or more pathogenic microbial agents.

Contagious disease: an infectious disease capable of being transmitted from one person to another.

Pathogen: a biological agent that causes disease also known as an infectious agent.

Body's Defences

- Skin
- Mucous Membranes
- Blood
- Inflammatory response
- Antibodies

Agents of Infectious Diseases

- Viruses
- Bacteria
- Fungi
- Protozoa / Arthropods
- Prions

Routes of Transmission

- Inhalation
- Digestion
- Inoculation
- Body Fluids
- Vectors

Prevention of Cross Infection

- Standard Precautions

  - Personal protective equipment
  - Decontamination
  - Sterilisation
  - Disposal of waste
  - Disposal of sharps
  - Single Use Items

Legislation affecting Infection Control:

- The Health Act 2006
- The Health and Safety at Work Act 1974
- Management of Health and Safety at Work Regulations 1999
- Control of Substances Hazardous to Health regulations 1988
- Environmental Protection Act 1990

National Initiatives to Control the Spread of Healthcare Acquired Infections

- NHS Decontamination Project 1999
- Winning Ways Guidelines (DH, 2003)
- Matrons Charter (NHS Estates, 2004)
- Towards Cleaner Hospitals (DH, 2004)
- Cleanyourhands Campaign (NPSA, 2004)
- Saving Lives Campaign (DH and NHS Modernisation Agency, 2005)

CHAPTER 2

Personal Protective Measures to Control Infection

Personal protective measures go far beyond the personal protective equipment mentioned in Standard Precautions (see Chapter 1). Personal protective measures protect the dental professional from any chance of becoming infected though contact with a patient, or of infecting a patient who they come into contact with before, during or after a visit to the dental surgery.

High standards of personal hygiene, both at work and at home, must be the norm for all dental professionals. Good habits should not be reserved for the dental surgery.

Immunisation

It is the dental nurses' responsibility to ensure immunity is maintained as part of their 'duty of care' under the Health and Safety at Work Act 1974, to protect themselves and anyone else they come into contact with. It is also part of the practice owners' duty of care, under the same Act, to ensure their staff are protected, thus safeguarding their patients' safety. The practice owner should keep records of their staffs' immunity and keep them up-to-date.

The DH (2006) gives four reasons as to why healthcare workers should be vaccinated against vaccine preventable diseases. These are:

- Protect individuals and their families from any occupationally acquired infection
- Protect patients and service users, including vulnerable patients who may not respond well to their own immunisation
- Protect other healthcare and laboratory staff
- Allow for efficient planning of services without disruption.

The starting point is effective immunisation against hepatitis B. All dental professionals should be immunised against hepatitis B, the only serious blood-borne infection that can, at present, be controlled by immunisation.

The immunity given by the three injection course should be checked by a blood test post-completion and thereafter by regular blood tests to check continued immunity. When necessary, immunity should be maintained by booster injections.

There is, at present, no effective immunisation against HIV/AIDS.

There is an increased incidence of pulmonary tuberculosis (TB) in the population and there are some that feel that healthcare professionals at risk should be immunised against this. Dental professionals are at risk from active TB infection as it is usually transmitted by droplet infection, coughing, sneezing, etc. It is recommended that unvaccinated tuberculin (negative individuals aged under 35 years) receive BCG (TB) vaccination (DH, 2006). There are no data available on the efficiency of protection afforded by BCG vaccination for those aged over 35 years and a clinical risk assessment should be carried out prior to vaccinating those ared over 35 years. BCG (TB) vaccination used to be routine for children before leaving school but is now risk-based and targeted at protecting children most at risk of exposure to TB. It is important to remember that TB can remain latent in individuals, who will carry the bacteria but show no symptoms.

Other infectious diseases should be taken into consideration by healthcare workers, including dental professionals. Patel (2007) warns of increasing danger to healthcare workers from the rise in cases of measles, mumps and rubella — diseases normally controlled by childhood vaccination — but a recent reduction in the uptake of the MMR vaccine has meant that once again we are seeing cases of these diseases. Patel (2007) advises that all healthcare workers should be up-to-date with their routine immunisations, such as tetanus, diphtheria, polio, measles, mumps and rubella. Dental professionals should also know their immunity to measles, rubella, and hepatitis B at all times so that should an outbreak occur then decisions can be made as to who is at risk. He also advises healthcare workers to take the opportunity to have the influenza vaccination if it is offered.

MRSA is not normally present in the oral cavity but it is possible to be occasionally isolated in oral infections. The British Dental Association (BDA, 2003) advises that any dentist or ancillary staff colonised by MRSA should not undertake or assist with invasive procedures. (The term 'colonisation' is used in the case of MRSA, instead of 'infection'). MRSA is often found in patients who have been discharged from hospital into the community. It colonises the nose, axillae and perineum and abnormal skin such as wounds, ulcers and eczematous skin.

Dental professionals, who cannot obtain immunity to hepatitis B by inoculation should not be excluded from working at the chairside, but such professionals should take extra care when handling contaminated instruments and waste. They should be scrupulous in their adherence to Standard Precautions.

Sharps and Needlestick Injury

Should any dental professional sustain a sharps or needlestick injury, the medical practitioner attending would need to know the immunisation status of the injured party.

The practice should have a written policy and procedure document on how to deal with such incidents, and all staff should be aware of its existence and follow it in the event of such an incident.

The policy/procedure should include the following:

- Wash the site thoroughly under running water
- Make the wound bleed if possible
- Seek medical advice immediately
    In general practice: immediate transfer to the A&E department of the nearest hospital
    In hospital or community clinic: follow the local infection control policy. This will often involve blood samples being taken from both the staff member and the patient to check the immunity levels of the staff and the infectivity of the patient. The incident should be reported to the occupational health department (OHD) immediately and the blood sample results sent to them. The OHD consultant will decide if further treatment is necessary
- If the patient is a known 'high risk' (i.e. a known hepatitis B or HIV/AIDS or hepatitis C carrier), precautionary action must be immediate and medical information about the patient should accompany the injured party to hospital so that reasoned decisions can be taken and informed advice given. If the decision is made that preventative treatment must be given, then a gammaglobulin injection must be administered within an hour, followed by a course of antiviral drugs
- There will have to be follow-up blood tests taken at the end of the course and at six months after the incident.

Patel (2007) reminds healthcare workers of their responsibilities under the Health and Safety at Work Act 1974 and that any instance of a healthcare worker contracting a vaccine-preventable infection must be reported by his or her employers, through the provision of the Health and Safety Executive and the Reporting of Injuries, Diseases and Dangerous Occurrences Regulations 1995 (DII, 1995). It may also be reportable as a serious untoward incident, to the Strategic Health Authority.

Hand Hygiene

One protective measure which forms an essential and primary component of standard precautions is effective hand hygiene. This should become second nature and be a standard procedure both in the clinical environment and in everyday life.

Ineffective hand hygiene has been identified as a significant contributory factor in the spread of healthcare acquired infections (HCAI). This was recognised by the National Patient Safety Agency (NPSA) when it launched its *Cleanyourhands* campaign (NPSA, 2004). The campaign was launched in 2004 in the acute hospital sector and involves the education and raising of awareness of staff, patients and visitors to the need for effective hand hygiene to help stop the spread of HCAIs. Washing hands effectively with soap and water can kill up to 95% of micro-organisms (NSPA, 2004). The campaign also advocated the use of alcohol hand-rubs by healthcare professionals and visitors. This resulted in alcohol hand-rub dispensers being placed at every bedside and at the entrance to wards and treatment rooms. Staff were encouraged to use alcohol hand-rubs before treating patients, and visitors were encouraged to use them when entering the ward or treatment area. Patients were also encouraged to question staff if they did not use the hand-rub. Alcohol hand-rubs are designed to be applied to visibly clean hands but must never be used as an alternative to washing contaminated hands. Nurses were encouraged to wash their hands more often, especially after treating a patient, changing dressings, etc.

In the dental care environment, where it is routine to wear rubber gloves, alcohol hand-rubs must never be used on examination gloves.

The need for effective hand hygiene has also been highlighted by National Institute for Clinical Excellence (NICE, 2003) and the British Medical Association (BMA, 2006).

Hand washing routine

An effective hand washing routine is illustrated in *Figure 1*. There are some basic rules which should be followed at all times. These include:

- Watches and stoned rings should be removed
- Nails should be kept short and no nail extensions worn
- Bracelets, friendship bands or other wrist jewelry should not be worn. If worn for religious reasons they must be pushed as far up the arm as possible and covered with tape
- If long sleeves are worn they must be able to be pushed up the arm to allow washing of the wrists
- Any broken skin or wounds should be covered with a waterproof dressing.

Effective hand washing should be performed in the following instances:

- When entering the surgery
- Before putting on gloves
- After removing gloves
- Before leaving the surgery
- After visiting the toilet
- Before and after handling food/drink
- After and before clearing up work area/handling instruments

Effective hand washing is checked by using an ultraviolet light box (see *Figures 2-4* overleaf). A specific lotion is applied to the hands and rubbed in the same way as soap would be used to wash the hands. The hands are then placed in the light box and the areas where the hands have been 'washed' effectively fluoresce blue. These are the areas covered by the lotion and would be washed effectively. Areas that do not fluoresce would not be washed effectively. The hands are then washed, using soap and water,

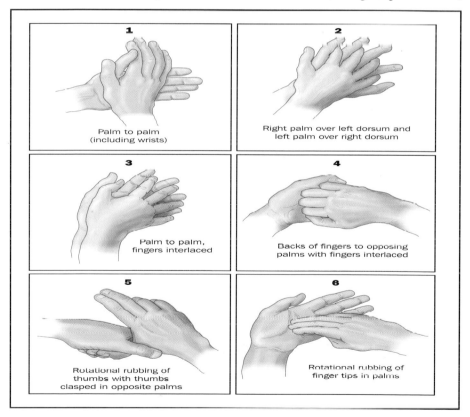

1

Palm to palm
(including wrists)

2

Right palm over left dorsum and
left palm over right dorsum

3

Palm to palm,
fingers interlaced

4

Backs of fingers to opposing
palms with fingers interlaced

5

Rotational rubbing of
thumbs with thumbs
clasped in opposite palms

6

Rotational rubbing of
finger tips in palms

Figure 1. Effective hand washing routine.

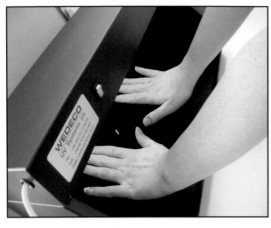

Figure 2. Hands coated in fluorescing lotion, under the UV light.

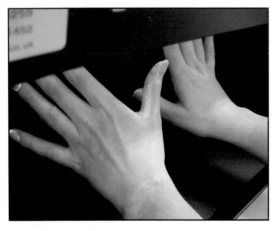

Figure 3. Hands after ineffective hand washing, showing that fluorescing lotion is still present.

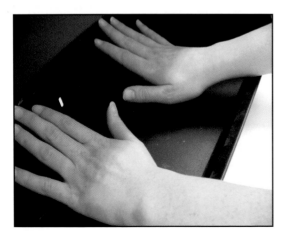

Figure 4. Hands after effective hand washing has removed all fluorescing lotion.

and again checked in the light box. Areas that still fluoresce have not been washed properly. This technique not only shows good hand washing practice but can also be used to assess effective surgical scrub techniques.

The hands illustrated in *Figure 3*, would still harbour micro-organisms in the areas fluorescing, as they had not been washed properly. The hands illustrated in *Figure 4*, would be 95% micro-organism free.

Getting into good habits when hand washing is an important tool in not only stopping the spread of infections but also in protecting yourselves against infections in the everyday environment. This should be only a part of impeccable personal hygiene. Frequent showers or baths, hair washing and clothes washing, as well as regular home cleaning, must be the norm and routine.

Personal Illness

Any scratches or abrasions must be covered by waterproof dressings. Dental professionals should take prompt action and advice if cuts or abrasions become infected, or if they become infected with diseases such as influenza or respiratory infections. Professionals who have conjunctivitis should not work as the condition is extremely contagious. If medical advice is sought the dental professional should let the doctor know what their job is and take advice as to whether or not to refrain from going to work.

It is commonly advised that, in an instance of diarrhoea and vomiting, an individual should not have been sick nor had diarrhoea for a clear 24 hours before returning to work. If a virulent infection of this nature is diagnosed then a clear 48 hours may be required before returning to work. If the infection continues then stool samples may need to be taken and submitted for investigation. In the case of any stomach upset, however severe or mild, good hand hygiene is of paramount importance in stopping the spread of the infection amongst others in the same environment.

Personal Protective Equipment

The provision and use of personal protective equipment (PPE) is governed by the Personal Protective Equipment at Work Regulations 1992 (DH, 1992) and its amendments up to 2002. The Regulations define PPE as:

'All equipment (including clothing affording protection against the weather) which is intended to be worn or held by a person at work and which protects them against one or more risks to their health and safety.'

DH, 1992

The regulations were drawn up and enacted as a direct consequence of the passing of the Health and Safety at Work Act 1974, which is the umbrella legislation covering all aspects of health and safety.

The main requirement of the regulations is that PPE is to be supplied and used at work wherever there are risks to health and safety that cannot be adequately controlled in other ways. It goes on to require that PPE:

- Is properly assessed before use to ensure suitability
- Is maintained and stored properly
- Is provided with instructions on how to use it safely
- Is used correctly by employees.

An employer cannot ask for money from an employee to pay for PPE, whether it is returnable or not. At the end of the employee's employment, they are expected to return any PPE as long as this fact is made clear in their contract of employment. If they fail to do so, then the employer may be able to deduct the cost of replacement from the final salary payment.

Before any PPE is bought, a risk assessment should be carried out to assess the suitability of any item bought. The following should be considered during the assessment:

- Is it appropriate for the tasks being undertaken and the risks involved with the task?
- Does it adequately control or prevent the risks without increasing the overall level of risk?
- Can it be adjusted to fit the wearer correctly?
- Has the health of the wearer been considered?
- What are the needs of the job and the demands placed on the wearer?
- Are the items of PPE compatible, if more than one item is to be worn or used at a time?

The areas at risk and the types of PPE needed are:

- Eyes: glasses, goggles, visors
- Head: helmets
- Breathing: filtering masks, respirators
- The body: overalls, uniforms
- Hands and arms: gloves, gauntlets
- Feet and legs: safety boots, leggings

It is also required that everyone using PPE must be trained in its use to:

- Raise awareness of the need for PPE, how and when it is used and its limitations
- Train and instruct staff in its correct use and set up systems to monitor compliance
- Ensure that users know that they must use the PPE whenever they are exposed to the risk, without exception, no matter for how short a time they are exposed
- Check that PPE is being worn and investigate any instances when PPE is not worn or used. Use posters to remind staff.

PPE must be maintained appropriately and stored correctly. It must be kept clean and in good repair and suitable replacements made available in the event of breakdown or failure.

The latest amendment to the regulations dated 2002 states that any PPE must have the 'CE' mark. This signifies that certain basic health and safety requirements have been met, which could involve testing and certification by an external body.

The regulations do not apply in certain cases when a risk is covered by a specific piece of health and safety legislation which demand the use of PPE as part of their requirements. The regulations of particular interest to the dental profession are:

- The Ionising Radiation Regulations 1999
- Control of Substances Hazardous to Health Regulations (as amended) 2002

Your practice should have a policy/document on the control of infection, and it should have a section devoted to the need, provision and use of PPE.

The BDA (2003) has a large section set aside to this subject and reiterates the need for immunisation as well as the use of PPE. It also points out the legal requirements placed on employing dentists, including that compliance should be written into a contract of employment.

The following sections discusse PPE with relevance to dentistry and dental professionals

Eyes

It is important that the eyes are protected from splatter and aerosols produced during dental treatment. Small fragments of amalgam, enamel, composite, calculus or other medicaments are sprayed out of the mouth during the use of rotary instruments and scalers, both mechanical and manual. The spray produced by airotors, cavitrons or airscalers is very fine and contains blood and saliva, either of which can carry pathogenic micro-organisms. The small fragments of material thrown out with the aerosol can cause damage to the sensitive tissues of the eye. Glasses should be worn at all times when working at the chairside. Fashion glasses do not give adequate protection and special PPE should be worn. Protective goggles or glasses should wrap around the face and be close-fitting. This will, however only protect the eyes and the use of visors to give whole face protection has become more common. Where prescription glasses are usually worn extra precautions must be taken to ensure complete protection, either by having prescription lenses put into wrap-around protective frames or by wearing goggles over the prescription glasses.

It is important to remember that the patient's eyes must also be protected from fragments and spray and also from the adverse effects of the use of UV curing lights. Some practices use tinted protective glasses for the patient but these do not give adequate protection against ultra violet light and the use of specially designed shields is imperative. It is also important to remember that the operator and chairside assistants' eyes must also be protected when using these lights.

Protective glasses, either used by operator, assistant or patient, must be thoroughly decontaminated after use. Those of the operator and assistant must be decontaminated after every patient to ensure no part can remain contaminated. This is best achieved by vigorous rubbing with alcohol wipes all over, including the side arms. The cheaper protective glasses become scratched very easily and will need to be replaced regularly. Any protective glasses contaminated, when used for a known infected patient, should be carefully cold sterilised. If this is not possible, then they should be disposed of in clinical waste. Manufacturer's instructions should be followed at all times.

Head

During normal dental procedures there is no need for head protection. However, this changes when surgical procedures are being carried out. During surgical procedures the head should be covered by a disposable paper cap to protect both operator and assistant from contamination by blood or saliva. There is not usually time to wash your hair between patients and there could be considerable contamination if aerosols have been created. The use of head protection also reduces any risk of anything in the hair, or the hair itself, contaminating the operative site. If using head caps they must be disposed of after single use and never reused.

Laboratory staff should take particular care with eye and nose protection because of the possibility of inhaling particles from items being prepared or trimmed, for example dentures and crowns. Risk assessments should be carried out as to the efficient removal of dust from grinding wheels and the handpieces used for trimming. It is possible to have screens fitted for technicians to work behind to protect their eyes, and position air suction systems alongside the work bench to remove dust, debris and fumes from materials.

Breathing

As with eye protection, operators and assistants can be affected by the aerosol created during operative dentistry procedures. Infected aerosols, fragments of materials and fragments of calculus can all be inhaled during such work.

It has been well documented that normal masks made of paper only give short-term, minimal protection. Recently, masks have been produced that contain a microbial filter and provide a much higher level of protection for a longer time. They are, naturally, much more expensive and there could be a temptation to use them more than once. Masks, of whichever type, are single use items and must be changed after every patient by both operator and assistant and never just pulled down to be reused.

The use of visors has become more commonplace recently, which give whole face protection and are often attached to protective wrap-around glasses. These visors do give better protection but at a higher cost and must only be used once, not simply wiped and reused. Visors have become popular for use when surgical procedures are being carried out as they protect the whole face from blood and saliva spatter.

Body

The body should be protected by the wearing of protective clothing, uniform, overalls, gowns or jackets. Any protective clothing used must be made of a material which can be machine washed at 65°C to ensure the eradication of potential contamination by micro-organisms.

The uniform should be practical for the purpose and it is commonly now made up of tunic and trousers rather than dresses for female dental nurses. Some practices promote a 'corporate image' by all staff wearing similar uniforms. The uniform should be clean each day and should not be worn outside the clinical environment. It is not good practice to wear a uniform on public transport since there is a high possibility of contamination arising, nor should it be worn to go to the shops during breaks.

The use of gowns to cover uniforms is recommended when surgical procedures are being carried out when there is a risk of significant blood contamination. It is possible to buy disposable, sterile gowns for such use but at a cost. Any fabric gown must be laundered at 65°C and on its own.

In some areas disposable plastic aprons are worn when an aerosol is being produced, but they provide little protection as not all the uniform is covered and should there be significant amounts of water this will run off the plastic surface.

There is no consensus on whether protective clothing should have long or short sleeves. There are positives and negatives for both: short sleeves allow effective hand washing, including wrists but leave the arms open to contamination by aerosol spatter. On the other hand, long sleeves protect arms from aerosol spatter contamination but make it impossible to effectively wash hands.

If a nurse or dentist is prone to eczema on the arms, then long sleeves will protect areas of broken skin from possible contamination.

Hands and arms

If arms are uncovered during operative procedures washing with soap and water before and at the end of treatment should be sufficient to protect against infection. However, any broken skin, wound, eczema or dermatitis should be protected by waterproof covers. Where eczema is extensive and ongoing then the wearing of long sleeves should be considered to ensure protection.

The care and protection of the hands is vital to infection control. Any broken skin offers an easy entry point for pathogens. The BDA (2003) recommends that gloves must be worn for all clinical procedures and treated as single use items, so a new pair of gloves must be used for each patient. Gloves should be donned immediately before contact with the patient and removed as soon as clinical treatment is complete. Used gloves must be disposed of in the clinical waste.

For the dental nurse, it is important to remember that they must not touch anything with contaminated gloves that cannot be sterilised. If there is a need to handle something the gloves must be removed and a fresh pair put on before continuing. Examination gloves must never be washed or rubbed with alcohol gel and reused.

Adams et al (1991) found that washing of gloves did not eradicate *Staphylococcus aureus* and that a significant proportion of gloves were found to be punctured. One major conclusion of the study was that rewashed gloves have the potential to cause cross–contamination. The study also concluded that lightweight examination gloves are far more prone to micropuncture formation than the heavier surgical type gloves. This is only one of many studies carried out on the decontamination of gloves, all of which prove that effective decontamination of rubber gloves is impossible and they must never be washed and worn for the treatment of a second or subsequent patient, by the dentist or any other dental professional. Gloves are designated 'single use' and as such if washed and reused lose their product liability, which passes to the user and could leave them open to litigation if cross-infection occurs.

When choosing gloves it is advisable to try differing makes as sizes will vary with manufacturer and the material used in their manufacture. You cannot rely on a 'small' glove made by one manufacturer being as good a fit as a 'small' glove made by another. The gloves should have textured fingertips to aid grip of small instruments, and they should come up to the wrist. Dental suppliers will often provide samples of the gloves available for staff to try and it should be remembered that what is a good fit for one person may not be as good for another.

Wearing gloves for long periods of time can be detrimental to the hands and it is advisable to follow some basic rules to protect your hands:

- Remove watches and stoned rings to facilitate effective washing up to and including the wrists
- Cover any broken skin, cuts or abrasions with waterproof dressings
- Perform effective hand washing as described previously
- Dry hands thoroughly using disposable paper towels
- Wash hands after removing gloves
- Regular use of a good emollient hand cream will help prevent skin drying out.

Although advisable to use an emollient hand cream regularly, care should be taken and manufacturers' information consulted as it is possible that some of the chemicals present in the hand cream can have a detrimental effect on the gloves. It is also possible that some dental materials can affect gloves and manufacturer's advice should be sought if there is any doubt. It has been known for some time that latex gloves have a detrimental effect on the setting times of some silicone impression material and in these cases non-latex gloves need to be worn by the nurse when mixing the putty phase.

Gloves chosen for use should comply with the European Standard BSEN 455 parts 1 and 2 — Medical Gloves for Single Use and carry the CE mark. They should always be powder free. Types of gloves available are:

- Non-sterile:
    Latex
    Vinyl
    Nitrile
    Hypoallergenic and low protein.

- Sterile:
    Latex
    Nitrile
    Hypoallergenic and low protein.

Sterile gloves are usually supplied in pairs, each pair individually wrapped and sterile until opened. They will have a shelf-life and should never be used after the use-by-date has passed as their sterility cannot be assured. Sterile gloves must always be worn by both the operator and assistant when carrying out sterile procedures. This is particularly important when undertaking implant surgery when the risk of infection and future failure must be reduced to an absolute minimum.

Non-sterile gloves are supplied in boxes of ambidextrous gloves as well as some being supplied in pairs. Again they will have a shelf life and if used beyond this will not guarantee the patency of the material.

Latex and Non-latex

More and more dental professionals are finding that latex gloves irritate their hands and there are now significant numbers of patients who have a latex sensitivity. For dental professionals who are latex sensitive or are developing irritant dermatitis the option of non-latex gloves is available,. These are usually made of a nitrile material. There are also gloves which a claim to be hypoallergenic or 'low protein'. It is imperative that the gloves purchased for dental professionals to wear are well fitting and of a material that is not irritant to their hands. There is a lot of different manufacturers who produce a whole range of different gloves — dental nurses in practice need to know that they do not have to put up with ill-fitting gloves that irritate them.

If the practice routinely uses latex gloves, then non-latex must be available for use on a latex-sensitive patient. Failure to do this could cause the patient to go into anaphylactic shock, which is potentially fatal. If latex gloves are routinely used, then special care must be taken before treating a latex-sensitive patient, not only with the type of glove used, but also the rubber dam and the local anaesthetic must have a latex-free bung. All surfaces must be very carefully cleaned as there could be residual latex dust on surfaces from the gloves.

However, there are disadvantages with non-latex gloves. Vinyl gloves tend to be thinner and may not be strong enough for extended use during longer procedures. Nitrile gloves are not as 'stretchy' as latex gloves and prove difficult to put on, especially if the hands are not dried thoroughly or if they are sweaty — the difficulty with putting on can lead to the gloves tearing. They can be supplied in strong colours which may be off putting to children or nervous patients. There is a new generation of non-latex gloves which are made from a nitrile type of material but have the stretchiness of latex. However, users have found they have adverse reactions to them where they do not have a reaction to nitrile. Some 'hypoallergenic' gloves are thicker and reduce tactile efficiency and are also supplied in pairs which can prove expensive if only one glove needs to be changed for any reason.

Dental nurses not only wear gloves at the chairside, but also when carrying out decontamination and sterilisation of instruments and equipment and also for general cleaning duties. Procedure gloves are not suitable for these activities; they are not thick enough to afford protection from puncture by sharp instruments or equipment. Heavy duty gloves should be used instead. Heavy duty gloves should be thick enough to resist puncture by sharp instruments but not so thick that they restrict movement of the fingers to perform the tasks. When handling any contaminated sharp instrument care and concentration are very important. Heavy duty gloves are reusable until they puncture, which may be in a short time.

Hand care

Care of the hands is essential. The constant washing of the hands and wearing of gloves is detrimental for the skin. It easily becomes dry and damaged and therefore open to infection. This can be alleviated to a certain extent by the use of a good quality liquid soap, with or without bactericide, thoroughly drying, using paper towels and the use of a good emollient cream. The soap should be in an elbow operated dispenser, to help prevent contamination. Any hand creams should have emollients in them to protect the skin. Highly perfumed 'hand creams' do not perform the same function and care should be taken to check that emollients do not adversely affect the material of the gloves worn — this information should be available from the manufacturers.

It is almost inevitable that, over a period of time, skin will become sensitive to the material of the gloves. It is rare for allergic contact dermatitis to develop, but should that happen, it could cause the person affected to cease practicing. Irritant contact dermatitis is more common and can be avoided by careful choice of gloves and meticulous hand care (BDA, 2003). If allergic contact dermatitis is suspected the advice of a specialist dermatologist should be sought.

Feet and Legs

Legs should be covered whenever working at the chairside for the same basic reasons why arms could be covered. This can be achieved by either wearing trousers or, for staff wearing dresses, tights or stockings. Having the feet and legs uncovered leaves them open to infection.

Professionals should give as much attention to their feet as they do to their hands. Attention should be paid to foot hygiene and nails. If athlete's foot is contracted or other infection or a verruca, then it should receive immediate attention and remedial treatment started. Nails should be kept short to avoid ingrowing toenails, which can lead to infections.

Shoes should be well-fitting with low or flat heels and completely enclose the foot, both toes and heels. It is advisable to wear leather shoes as leather is breathable and will help with problems of excessive perspiration. Shoes should be comfortable, and although dental professionals sit at the chairside now and not stand as many years ago, the footwear will be worn for nine or more hours. A nurse with sore feet will not be concentrating on the job and they will be fidgeting to try and make their feet comfortable. In the event of a medical emergency there may be a need to run to get equipment therefore high heels are not suitable. The soles of the shoes should be of a non-slip material as water on the floor is an ever present problem in the dental surgery.

Toes should be covered to help eliminate, as far as possible, any chance of injury from dropped instruments or equipment. It is as much a sharps injury if your toe is stabbed by a contaminated instrument, as it is if your finger is stabbed.

Finally, do not forget that there is also a duty of care on the part of dentists to ensure that items sent to laboratories are decontaminated and evidence sent with the item to confirm this. This is also true for items of equipment sent to external repair companies.

References

Adams et al (1992) A clinical evaluation of glove washing and re-use in dental practice. *Journal of Hospital Infection* **120:** 153–62

BDA (2003) *Infection Control in Dentistry: Advice Sheet A12.* British Dental Association, London

BMA (2006) *Healthcare Associated Infections — A Guide for Healthcare Professionals*: British Medical Association, London

CDC (2005) *Oral Health Resources — Infection Control — Frequently Asked Questions.* Centre for Disease Control, London

DH (2006) *Immunisation Against Infectious Disease.* HMSO, London

DH (2000) *Ionising Radiation Regulations 1999 and subsequent amendments 2000.* HMSO, London

DH (1995) *Reporting of Injuries, Diseases and Dangerous Occurrence Regulations 1995 (RIDDOR).* HMSO, London

DH (1992) *Personal Protective Equipment at Work regulations 1992.* HMSO, London

DH (1988) *Control of Substances Hazardous to Health (COSHH) Regulations 1988.* HMSO, London

DH (1974) *Health and Safety at Work Act 1974.* HMSO, London

NICE (2003) *Infection Control. Prevention of Healthcare Associated Infection in Primary and Community Care.* NICE, London

NPSA (2004) *Cleanyourhands Campaign.* National Patient Safety Agency, London

Patel B (2007) Immunisation of healthcare workers update. *British Journal of Infection Control* **8**(3): 63

CHECKLIST 2

Immunisation

- Hepatitis B
- HIV / AIDS
- Tuberculosis
- Measles, Mumps and Rubella
- MRSA Colonisation

Hand Hygiene

- Hand Washing Technique
- Hand Care

Personal Protective Equipment

- Personal Protective Equipment at Work Regulations 1992
- Ionising Radiation Regulations 1999
- Control of Substances Hazardous to Health Regulations 1988

At-Risk Areas

- Eyes
- Head
- Breathing
- The Body
- Hands and Arms
- Feet and Legs

Equipment

- Goggles
- Masks
- Uniform
- Gloves
- Shoes

CHAPTER 3

Surgery Preparation and Maintenance

The preparation and maintenance of the dental surgery and total dental environment is fundamental to effective compliance with Standard Precautions and therefore to infection control in general. The total environment has to be decontaminated, maintained and cleaned effectively to assist with infection control procedures. Infection control does not and cannot begin and end with only instrument care.

Good design and layout is the basis for competent decontamination and infection control. Dust and debris collect in inaccessible places, particularly corners and joins in flooring and work surfaces. Most dental nurses go to work in a practice that is already set up and cannot influence the design or the equipment used. However, where there is an opportunity for nurses and other professionals to have a say in the design and equipping of a new surgery or practice, they should do so. The BDA (2003) gives detailed advice about the planning of surgeries, ventilation, floor covering, work surfaces, the choice of equipment and the impact on utilities (for example water).

When planning a new surgery or refurbishing an existing facility, the following points should be taken into consideration:

- Its ease of use
- Its operational efficiency
- Ease of implementation of infection control procedures.

These will be influenced by certain factors:

- The size and shape of the area
- The types and positions of fixtures
- Type and position of the dental chair and unit
- Type and position of accessory equipment.

There should be space for staff to work in optimum positions and there should be room for mobile equipment to be moved around and used easily and efficiently. Consideration should be given for space for wheelchairs and the access to the surgery being wheelchair accessible.

Basic Needs for a Dental Surgery

- There should be two distinct areas in the surgery, one for the dentist and one for the dental nurse
- Each should have a hand wash basin which should have elbow or foot operated taps and liquid soap dispensers
- The dentist's side should have access to handpieces, triple air syringe, bracket table where fitted, and light
- The nurse's side should have access to the aspirator lines, triple air syringe, curing light and materials
- The nurse's side should also have access to clinical waste disposal bins and a space for contaminated equipment to be processed
- Clean and dirty areas should be clearly defined
- Dirty instruments should, where possible, be decontaminated in a separate area which also contains the equipment to decontaminate and sterilise them
- The decontamination area should have a separate hand wash basin from the decontamination sink
- If mechanical decontamination is not used, the decontamination sink must be deep enough to allow total immersion of the instruments during cleaning.

Ventilation

- The surgery should be well ventilated using an opening window but with a fan available when this is inappropriate
- Any systems used should exhaust to the outside, ensuring there is no risk to people passing by or other buildings
- There are recommended rates of supply of fresh air and these should be considered when choosing a system
- Any mechanical system installed must be able to be cleaned easily to eliminate the risk of the system circulating micro-organisms and pathogens
- It is not recommended to install recycling air conditioning systems.

Floor Coverings

- It is essential that the covering is impervious and non-slip

- Carpeting in the surgery is to be avoided, but may be appropriate for waiting areas
- The covering should be seam free, but where there are seams, they must be sealed
- The junctions between floor and wall or between floor and cabinetry should be 'coved' or sealed to prevent inaccessible areas which are impossible to clean.

Work Surfaces

- Work surfaces should be impervious and smooth and easy to clean and disinfect
- As far as possible they should be joint-free, but where there are joins they must be sealed to stop debris collecting in them
- All junctions should be curved or rounded to allow effective cleaning.

Choice of Equipment

When choosing new equipment there are certain points that should be taken into consideration:

- Is the equipment fit for the purpose you intend to use it for?
- Is it compatible with other equipment in the surgery that you are not replacing?
- Its ease of use and maintenance
- Does it have a CE mark to demonstrate compliance with Medical Devices Regulations? (BDA, 2003; HPRA, 2003)
- How easy is it to follow the manufacturer's decontamination recommendations?
- New instruments with serrated handles are difficult to clean effectively
- Instruments with hinges pose a potential problem for effective cleaning
- Check the manufacturer's instructions about the cleaning of the fabric of a new dental chair; will it be detrimental to disinfect it regularly and cause the fabric to deteriorate?
- Is there a foot control option on equipment?
- What training is necessary to use it safely?

Water Supplies

It is imperative that the quality of the water coming through a dental unit is as pure as possible since dental professionals and patients are regularly exposed to water and aerosols produced during dental treatment.

The microbial contamination of dental water lines was studied by Pankhurst et al (1998). The paper studied the build up of biofilms on the periphery of unit waterlines, where flow is at its minimum, and the intermittent use of lines, leading to stagnation of water in them. Biofilms build up inside these lines and they are more difficult to remove than free-flowing microbes. The paper goes on to advocate the use of anti-retraction valves and removable filters and a robust regime of flushing at the start of every day. Although flushing has no effect on the biofilms that are present, it will remove stagnant and potentially contaminated water from the lines. For larger institutions and buildings (for example dental hospitals) the use of chlorination in higher doses is recommended to help eliminate microbes particularly Legionella, but it recognise that there is increasing resistance to this process by the bacteria (Pankhurst et al, 1998). Other recommendations include that flushing through water lines between patients and at the beginning and end of the working day is a useful method to eliminate oral flora entering the waterlines via suck-back. The Health and Safety Executive (HSE, 2001) published a revised approved code of practice on the control of Legionella in water systems.

It is important that all local regulations concerning use of water and sewerage systems are consulted and the local water and sewerage provider consulted before substances are emitted into the waste systems. This should be checked at regular intervals and advice sought if regulations change. This action should be taken before a new dental surgery is set up to avoid problems:

- Water lines should be fitted with anti-retraction valves to help eliminate contamination
- Dental unit water lines are known to harbour biofilms, which can be a source of Legionella bacteria
- Some newer dental units use a reservoir bottle for the water supply instead of being connected to mains water
- Bottled water can have disinfectants added to reduce the microbial load
- Check if the equipment has an air-gap to assist with preventing contamination of the water supply by backflow from equipment used.

Sinks should be designated as 'hand wash only' and 'decontamination only'. The decontamination sink should be used to put put items before transfer to the decontamination area, if there is a separate area. If there is no separate area, then this sink should be deep enough to allow the items to be totally immersed during decontamination. It should not be used for hand washing. Where a separate decontamination area is provided, careful selection of the equipment for it is essential. A decision has to be made whether to install an ultrasonic cleaner and which type and size is best, or a washer/disinfector. A suitable autoclave must be chosen. This equipment will be discussed in a later chapter.

Ideally there should be a separate area within the surgery for administration purposes, the writing up of patient's notes etc. This area could contain a computer, if the practice is computerised for patient records, digital radiographs, etc. There should also be an area set aside for the taking of radiographs, complete with all the necessary screening and safety equipment.

Consideration should also be given to any extra precautions and standards that are required if surgical work is to be carried out (for example implants), or if patients are to be treated under conscious sedation or inhalation sedation — the latter requiring an active scavenging system to be installed.

With so much to be considered it is no surprise to know that there are a growing number of specialist designers for dental surgeries and practices, not least among them the equipment manufacturing companies.

Procedures

Once the surgery is built and equipped and before it is put to regular use all the staff must receive competent training on all the new equipment installed and must be completely happy with its safe use, decontamination, maintenance and storage. For professionals working in the hospital or private dental service, there will be training made available for new employees and there will be policies and procedures in place for the decontamination of equipment and the procedures to be followed before, between and after patient treatment. These policies must be adhered to at all times. All new members of staff should have an induction into these policies and procedures as well as training where necessary. It should be documented that copies of the policy have been given to new staff and also documented that adequate and appropriate training has been given. Staff should also sign to say that they have received these.

The procedures outlined below are general procedures and must not be used in place of agreed policies, unless agreed by the practice owner.

Surgery Preparation at the Start of the Day

To comply with the needs of Standard Precautions, the whole surgery area must be considered as 'contaminated' or liable to contamination. Therefore the whole area must be decontaminated at the start of every day:

- Ensure that all devices are switched on (compressor, suction apparatus, dental chair and unit, accessory equipment) where appropriate
- Put on protective clothing to cover the uniform (plastic apron, heavy duty rubber gloves and protective goggles)
- If appropriate all water lines should be flushed through for a few minutes. This is not necessary if a bottle reservoir is used in the unit as in this case it will only be necessary to ensure the water is coming through from the reservoir, when first filled. Wear a mask to do this to prevent inhalation of any aerosol produced
- All water lines on the unit, handpiece tubings, triple air syringe tubings, spittoon and tumbler filler, must be run through to allow chemicals in the water to destroy any microbes. This can include the potentially deadly Legionella bacteria. This should be done before any wiping down, as an aerosol is produced which would contaminate any previously decontaminated area
- Make up fresh detergent and disinfectant solutions to manufacturers' instructions
- Clean all surfaces of the dental chair and unit, work surfaces and accessory equipment with a detergent solution
- Wipe all the above surfaces with a disinfectant capable of killing viruses, bacteria and fungi
- When all cleaning has been completed remove protective glasses, plastic apron, heavy duty gloves, mask and glasses. Put disposable items in the clinical waste
- Put on a clean pair of examination gloves and 'lay up' the surgery
- The amount of decontamination needed between patients will be greatly reduced if a rigorous 'zoning' system is employed by both dentist and nurse
- Prepare a 'dirty' zone by covering the surface with an impermeable cover or whatever the infection control policy requires. This is any area that will receive a contaminated item, for example the bracket table
- Cover light handles and chair controls, if not foot operated,

with an impermeable sheet. These sheets are available on a roll and are suitable for protecting tubing, triple syringe handles and other unsterilisable items attached to the dental unit

- Areas that will remain 'clean' can be covered by a disposable paper cover
- When all areas have been covered appropriately put out the equipment and instruments ready for the first treatment
- Do not put out anything that is not certain to be used. Keep items that may be required away from the 'dirty' zone but readily available if needed
- Put out any disposable items, for example aspirator tubes, saliva ejectors, triple syringe tips, cups
- Medicaments that are required during treatment should be kept in the 'clean' area and handled carefully so as not to contaminate them
- The patient's treatment notes should be kept away from the operative area so as to avoid possible contamination.
- An increasing number of practices use computers for recording treatment, chartings and digital radiographs. The monitors and computers and other peripherals should be kept away from possible contamination and form part of the decontamination procedure
- Care should be taken when wiping over computer equipment, especially the keyboard. It is possible to purchase covers for computer keyboards to assist with effective decontamination
- Care and thought should be taken before using the computer mouse to avoid contamination from gloves
- When the surgery is ready the decontamination room or area must be prepared. The ultrasonic cleaner should be filled with water and a suitable enzymatic cleaner or the washer/disinfector prepared according to manufacturers' instructions. The autoclave should be filled with deionised water and tested. A fuller description of these processes will be given in a later chapter
- Check that all and any items that are required for the treatment session are available. Good planning and a robust ordering system are essential to the efficient working of a treatment session.

Decontamination Between Patients

When the treatment is finished and the patient has left the surgery it must be decontaminated before the next patient is brought in. It is at this time that the nurse will appreciate successful zoning. The only areas that have to be cleaned and disinfected are the ones that have been contaminated by dirty instruments, handpieces, etc. An experienced and efficient nurse will work in such a way as to minimise contamination and will clear as they work:

- Using heavy duty gloves remove all contaminated instruments, papers, handpieces and accessory equipment and put in the decontamination room or in the designated decontamination sink
- Put all disposables into the clinical waste bag
- Put any 'sharps' (needles, burs, matrix bands, endo syringes, etc) into an appropriate sharps container
- Remove any disposable impermeable covers and put into the clinical waste
- Run water through the handpiece and triple air syringe tubings for 20–30 seconds to eliminate contamination due to backflow/back-syphonage
- Aspirate some clean water through the aspirator tubing
- Clean all contaminated areas with detergent solution followed by an appropriate disinfectant with viricidal, bactericidal and fungicidal properties
- Disinfect any unsterilisable items such as protective glasses
- Put on fresh examination gloves and put out fresh covers and disposable items, followed by all the equipment and instruments needed for the next procedure
- Ideally, another person should decontaminate the used items as the dental nurse will be fully occupied with the next patient
- If no other person is available, the nurse must evolve systems of working to do both essential duties effectively and efficiently
- In a multi-dentist practice systems must be organised and arranged between all nurses to perform the decontamination and sterilisation of contaminated items.

Decontamination at the End of the Session

After the last patient for the session has left the surgery, follow the previous procedure to clear the contaminated area. In addition, the following must be carried out:

- All 'clean' zones must be cleaned with detergent solution followed by an appropriate disinfectant. Wear protective glasses as well as gloves to prevent splashes getting into the eyes
- The surgery should be well ventilated at this stage to help dispel

any harmful fumes

- Disinfect any items to be sent to the laboratory and complete the appropriate disinfection certificate and put ready for collection or posting
- Any items for repair should also be disinfected and prepared for collection or posting, with the appropriate disinfection certificates completed
- If this break is only short (for example lunch), then the surgery can be 'laid up' ready for the next session
- If this is the end of the day then there are further decontamination processes that must be followed and which are explained below.

Decontamination at the End of the Day

- Follow the procedure for the 'end of the session' outlined above
- All accessory equipment should be put away after being thoroughly wiped with disinfectant or an alcohol wipe, depending on manufacturers' instructions
- All electrical accessory equipment should be unplugged and stored away
- The computer should be closed down and turned off at the mains and then wiped down with disinfectant or alcohol wipes
- All work surfaces and equipment must be cleaned with detergent followed by a suitable disinfectant
- If the unit uses bottled water the bottle should be emptied and disinfected following manufacturers' instructions
- Some policies call for the use of a bleach solution, sodium hypochlorite, at a concentration of 1000 parts per million for basic disinfection. For blood spillages, a concentration of 10,000 parts per million. If used, this should be allowed to lie on surfaces for up to 30 minutes
- Aspirators must be run through with a suitable disinfectant, again according to manufacturers' instructions. This will help to break down any biofilms which can form in the tubing. The disinfectant used must be non-foaming, household detergent will not suffice. A foaming solution will damage the suction equipment
- Some of the newer dental units have built in disinfection systems for handpiece tubing, spittoon and aspiration. If available these systems should be used to ensure effective disinfection of the unit

- If a portable suction unit is used it is very difficult, if not impossible, to effectively clean and disinfect the mechanism, and disposal of the contents poses a considerable hazard. They also do not contain any filters. For these reasons, the use of portable suction equipment is not recommended
- Any local regulations for the disinfection of drains or drainage systems must be followed to the letter
- All clinical waste should be prepared for collection in line with local regulations and arrangements
- All used instruments and contaminated equipment should be sterilised and stored in clean dry receptacles. No contaminated instruments should be left overnight; they pose a risk to anyone coming into the surgery
- When the surgery has been completely decontaminated and closed down the decontamination area must also be cleaned and closed down.
- Ultrasonic baths have to be unplugged, emptied, cleaned out and dried
- Washer/disinfectors must be cleaned and closed down according to manufacturers' instructions
- Autoclaves should be drained, turned off and unplugged
- All other surfaces and any other decontamination equipment should be cleaned down with detergent followed by disinfectant
- Before leaving the surgery check that all windows are closed and all equipment turned off and unplugged and left in a safe manner.

During the process of decontamination, at any time, the nurse should wear protective clothing, plastic aprons, glasses, mask and appropriate gloves, removing contaminated items and replacing with clean whenever appropriate. Gloves should be changed after cleaning and before handling clean items. Hands should be washed when entering the surgery first thing in the morning and any time before leaving the surgery and certainly when leaving finally at the end of the day.

Maintenance of Equipment

The preparation of the surgery at the start of the day, between patients and at the end of the session or day, is different to the maintenance required to keep equipment working at optimum efficiency and to forestall breakdowns. Comprehensive schedules of maintenance by outside engineers should be kept and followed. Failure to have routine maintenance carried out could lead to breakdowns thereby inconveniencing both the dental team and the patient. The basic advice for the maintenance of any equipment is to follow the manufacturer's instructions at all times. Failure to follow these instructions will invalidate the warranty.

Handpieces are particularly vulnerable to breakdown if not maintained correctly. Unless otherwise advised by the manufacturer, they should be oiled before autoclaving. If advised, oil immediately after autoclaving, but run through briefly to disperse any excess oil. If some handpieces are oiled before autoclaving whilst some are oiled after, then two different oiling devices must be used to avoid contamination of the sterilised items. It is possible to buy machines which will automatically clean, oil and sterilise handpieces, ensuring that the lumen inside the handpiece is completely decontaminated and sterilised. Special procedures have to be followed before disinfecting handpieces in washer/disinfectors, and it is essential that the manufacturer's instructions for both the handpiece and the washer/ disinfector are followed strictly.

Attention must be paid to the tips of light curing lights. It is easy for them to become coated with either bonding solution or composite during use. If either are allowed to build up the efficiency of the light is impaired and the material being cured will not be cured properly, which could lead to failure of the filling. Light tips should be cleaned thoroughly after use and tested regularly to ensure sufficient light is being emitted. Many curing lights have a test gauge attached, but if not there are test gauges available for purchase.

If inhalation sedation (IS) — previously known as relative analgesia — (RA) is carried out in the surgery routine maintenance of the equipment is essential. If this is allowed to lapse then a patient's life could be put at risk. Gauges have to be checked to be sure they give correct information about flow rates and cylinder contents. The emergency oxygen button must always be working efficiently. The scavenging system operating in the surgery must also be regularly checked and maintained to ensure staff are not put at risk from exhausted anaesthetic gases. It is possible to purchase monitors which will record levels of N_2O in the atmosphere where IS is being used.

The same is also true of pulse oximeters and other equipment used when patients are given intravenous sedation, and for emergency equipment kept in case of medical emergency.

General Cleaning

Maintenance also includes cleaning. Cleaning of equipment and surgery fixtures and fittings must be recognised as maintenance. Cleaning schedules should be prepared in consultation with all staff as they must be relevant to all areas of the practice, not just the surgery. There is little point in keeping the surgery spotless and as infection-free as possible if the waiting area is thick with dust and the toilet is not kept clean. Pathogens can be carried from one area to another and will not stop at the surgery door.

There should be cleaners employed to clean 'public' areas and other areas as agreed but these cleaners should also have training in the requirements of infection control and their responsibilities towards its effective implementation.

Toilets should be cleaned daily and paper towels and liquid soap replenished as soon as required.

Any staff rooms or the kitchen should be cleaned regularly and no food allowed to be kept past its 'use by date'. Fridges should be regularly wiped out and, where necessary, defrosted. It is essential that food and medicines or drugs are not stored in the same fridge as it is possible for food to be contaminated with the contents of packets of medicaments or drugs and vice versa.

Dirty laundry should not be allowed to lie about in staff areas; it should always be placed in a designated 'dirty' area immediately after use.

The office area should be dusted and, if carpeted, vacuumed regularly. Vacuum cleaners must never be used in the surgery as they exhaust possible pathogen-contaminated air.

Computer equipment, whether in the office, reception desk or surgery, will attract dust by static attraction and must be decontaminated daily. The reception desk should be dusted and uncluttered. Health education leaflets in holders should be kept tidy and the holders dusted daily.

The floor in the surgery should be covered with a non-slip covering, not carpet as it is impossible to decontaminate carpet in a surgery. Bacteriostatic floor coverings are now available, but at extra cost. The floor of the surgery should be cleaned every day and the walls wiped down regularly, using a disinfectant. Particular attention must be given to any seams in the flooring as they can become reservoirs for dust, debris and pathogens. Floor coverings taken a few inches up the wall will make cleaning considerably easier than if there is a junction between floor and wall.

Cupboards and storage areas should be cleaned regularly and materials stored in them checked for 'use by dates' and to ensure correct rotation of presterilised items and packed sterile instruments.

This total cleaning package is not the responsibility of the dental nurse. Cleaners should be employed to clean 'public' areas, but specialist equipment must be the responsibility of the dental nurse. This will ensure correct cleaning regimes and correct solutions are used. However, this is only possible if the nurse is trained correctly and this training is the responsibility of the dentist or practice manager.

The nurse should be involved in discussions with suppliers of new equipment when it is fitted to ascertain correct cleaning and maintenance regimes are followed.

The dental nurse should check that cleaning is carried out effectively and efficiently and not be afraid to report poor practices. The dental nurse should demonstrate high standards of cleaning and infection control in their areas and should insist on the same standards being maintained in other areas of the practice.

Detailed systems, policies and procedures for the preparation and maintenance of the dental surgery are essential to the overall infection control regime.

References

BDA (2003) *Infection Control in Dentistry: Advice Sheet A12*. BDA, London

HSE (2001) *Legionnaires' Disease: The Control of Legionella Bacteria in Water Systems — revised Approved Code of Practice LA 01/2001*. HSE, London

MHRA (2003) *Medical Devices (Amendment) Regulations 2003 – SI 2003/1697*. Medicines and Healthcare Products Regulatory Agency, London

Pankhurst CL, Johnson NW, Woods RG (1998) Microbial contamination of dental unit waterlines: the scientific argument. *International Dental Journal* **48:** 359–68

CHECKLIST 3

Design and Layout

- General advice
- Ventilation
- Floor Coverings
- Choice of Equipment
- Water Supplies

Preparation at the start of the day

- Turning on equipment
- Flushing water lines through
- Cleaning and disinfecting all surfaces
- Preparing accessory equipment
- Covering and zoning the area
- Putting out disposable items
- Putting out equipment for first patient
- Preparing the decontamination room/area

Between patients

- Clearing contaminated zone
- Cleaning and disinfecting contaminated zone
- Removing contaminated items to decontamination room/area
- Running through water lines and suction
- Recovering contaminated zone
- Putting out sufficient equipment for the next patient

At the end of the Session

- Clear as for between patients
- Clean and disinfect all areas, even those not contaminated
- Decontaminate and fill in certificate for any items to go to the laboratory
- Decontaminate and fill in certificate for any items requiring repair
- Lay out equipment for first patient of next session, if at lunchtime

At the end of the day

As at the end of a session
- Clean and disinfect all areas and equipment
- Wipe down any accessory equipment
- Put as much equipment away in cupboards as possible
- Sterilise all contaminated instruments, handpieces, etc.
- Do not leave any contaminated items, putting others at risk
- Collect up all clinical waste and put ready for collection
- Follow local regulations for water lines, waste, etc.
- Ensure all decontamination equipment is emptied or drained
- Close computer down and turn off at mains
- Ensure all equipment is turned off at the mains or unplugged
- Close windows and turn off lights

During all preparation and clearing

Be aware of the risk of contamination caused by not changing gloves
and other protective clothing during all stages.

Maintenance of Equipment

- Follow manufacturer's instructions
- Rigorous and comprehensive maintenance schedules
- Handpiece oiling and sterilisation
- Curing light efficiency.
- Inhalation Sedation Equipment
- Special equipment for conscious sedation
- Medical emergency equipment

Cleaning

- Cleaning schedules
- All areas must be as clean as the surgery
- Areas of responsibility
- Nurses responsibility
- Insistence on high standards throughout the practice

CHAPTER 4

Care and Maintenance of Instruments and Equipment

All instruments and equipment, as well as many other items, used in the dental surgery are classed as Medical Devices. The NHS Executive sent a letter in 1998 which outlined the changes in legislation (Department of Health [DH], 1998). It went on to define a medical device as:

'An instrument, apparatus, appliance, material or other article, whether used alone or in combination, together with any software necessary for its proper application which:

a) is intended by the manufacturer to be used for human beings for the purpose of:

    i.   *diagnosis, prevention, monitoring, treatment or alleviation of disease*

    ii.   *diagnosis, monitoring, treatment, alleviation of or compensation for an injury or handicap*

    iii.   *investigation, replacement or modification of anatomy or a physiological process, or*

    iv.   *control of conception, and*

b)   *does not achieve its principal intended action in or on the human body by pharmacological, immunological or metabolic means, even it is assisted in its function by such means.'*

DH, 1998

In simple terms, this means that any instrument, item of equipment or accessory to these is classified as a medical device and as such is controlled by the Medical Devices Directives and Regulations (Healthcare Products Regulatory Agency [MHRA], 1993, 1994, 2002).

With effect from June 1998, all medical devices must have a 'CE' mark (DH, 1998). This mark shows that the item has been manufactured to high standards and that it complies with health and safety requirements. This was outlined in a Medical Devices Directive (MHRA, 1993) and implemented into UK law by the Medical Devices Regulations (MHRA, 1994, 2002). These regulations were revised in 2002 and updated in 2006:

This whole raft of legislation is enacted with the express purpose of safeguarding the public and the user from inferior products which could fail, with serious consequences. It covers everything that is used in the dental surgery. When any new pieces of equipment or instruments are bought the item should be checked to ensure it has the 'CE' mark. If it does not then very serious consideration must be given as to whether the item is fit for the purpose it is being purchased for. Other considerations must be investigated before purchasing a new item include:

- Is it compatible with other equipment already in place and which is not being changed?
- If the new item is not compatible with existing equipment, it could mean the purchase of extra accessory equipment. For example, if a new light curing lamp is to be bought, will the existing tips fit it?
- Is the item fit for the purpose it is being bought for?
- Does the item do the job completely, or does it need extras bought to make it work?
- What extra training is required for the correct use of the item?
- Will any extra training required impact on the equipment being put into immediate use?
- Who will deliver that training and will it impact on when the item can be put into use?
- How will it impact on the health and safety of its users?
- Are there any manual handling problems connected to it?
- Is there a need to purchase any other safety equipment or personal protective equipment?
- Will it have a detrimental impact on the surrounding environment?
- Does it create any issues as to waste or other environmental areas, such as fumes or dust emission?
- Will the waste management arrangements have to be altered to accommodate the equipment and its use?
- Is it value for money? Cheapest is not necessarily best
- Does it really do what is needed or has it just been chosen because it is the cheapest?
- Is the maintenance and everyday care of the item within the capabilities of the user?
- Will the user/maintainer need specific training to maintain it which is beyond their experience and outside their job description?

There may be other considerations to be taken into account by laboratory owners when purchasing new equipment. These could include whether or not the equipment requires active air evacuation of dust and where this would be evacuated to.

There are also serious considerations to be made when using some materials, for example, the fumes from acrylic monomers can contain methyl methacrylate which, in great concentrations, can be carcinogenic. Other considerations may be the placing of a porcelain 'oven' because of the heat emitted during use and what precautions are necessary for the user of handpieces or polishing wheels to adjust and polish dentures or crowns because of the dust created.

The overriding advice with any new piece of equipment or instrument, when it comes to its care and maintenance is to follow the manufacturer's instructions and advice. Failure to take this advice will lead to the guarantee or warranty being invalidated and it would be wise to check if there are restrictions placed on its maintenance or repair. The guarantee, or warranty, may require maintenance to be carried out at set intervals and by registered technicians along with repair being carried out in the same way. It is essential that the practice or clinic has rigorous maintenance regimes set up and adhered to.

The organisation of maintenance schedules is the responsibility of the practice owner, or in the case of hospitals or PDS clinics, the manager in charge. It is not the responsibility of dental nurses to set up these arrangements, but it is their responsibility to report any problems with equipment and check that schedules are being followed.

Care and Maintenance of Hand Instruments

Some hand instruments need no other care and maintenance other than effective cleaning. An experienced dental nurse will wipe materials and other debris from instruments before it is allowed to set during the treatment — caution must be taken not to have a sharps injury whilst carrying this out.

However, there are a number of groups of hand instruments which require regular and specific maintenance other than just cleaning.

Mouth Mirrors
Mouth mirrors are supplied as a handle with a separate, usually screw-in, head. The handle needs no more care than effective cleaning, but the head will become scratched, fogged or covered with materials during normal use. This will make it unusable and the head should be removed, placed in a 'sharps bin' and replaced with a new one. This is something which the person carrying out

decontamination and sterilisation should be aware of and should check the state of mirror heads at regular intervals, if not at every use. There are different sizes of mirror head, smaller ones for use with children or patients with limited opening and larger ones for everyday use. It is also possible to buy 'front surface' mirror heads which give a clearer image. These are particularly useful when carrying out endodontic procedures or advanced restorative work. It is the dentist who must decide which size and type of mirror is required and the person changing it to ensure the correct new one is fitted.

Some orthodontic practices use photographic mirrors during treatment which may require different decontamination procedures. These are often fitted into a special handle which has a slot to receive the head rather than a screw thread.

Probes (other than periodontal or CPITN probes)
Right angle, contra-angled and sickle probes are sharp and need to be so. They are used to check for caries and crown preparation margins, etc. and need to have a sharp, fine point to do so. Over time, with repeated use, cleaning and sterilisation, they will become blunt and ineffective. It is possible to sharpen probes so that they retain their fine point, however if carried out over a long period, the probe will become shorter and unusable and will need to be replaced. This fact should not deter the dentist from insisting that they have a sharp probe to use.

They can be sharpened manually or using an electric wheel.

Excavators
Whatever size or whether angled or straight, they need to be sharp to be effective in their use for removing caries. They are also used for the removal of granulation tissue and other tissue during surgical procedures. They will, as with probes, lose their edge with use and sterilisation and need to be sharpened regularly.

Carvers, chisels and cervical margin trimmers
These all need to have a sharp edge to be effective in their use and will need sharpening at intervals, depending on use.

Hand scalers
These cannot perform their task of removing calculus unless they have a sharp, fine edge. They will need sharpening at very frequent intervals, depending on use. The very nature of the instrument, having different cutting edges and angles, makes their sharpening very important. If a scaler is sharpened at the wrong angle or along the wrong edge it will be almost useless and will need replacing.

Many hygienists and therapists use cushioned grip handled scalers. This overcomes the ergonomic problems of using fine movements and gripping fine handled instruments for long periods of time. If a hygienist is employed in a practice or where they are employed in hospitals or clinics they will undertake the sharpening of their own scalers, but where they are not employed, then someone else must take on the responsibility. It is imperative that the person is fully trained and totally competent in doing this otherwise it could be extremely costly in terms of replacement instruments having to be bought.

A natural consequence of repeated sharpening of scalers, is that the tips become extremely thin and brittle. Whoever sharpens the scalers must be aware of this and alert when carrying out the sharpening and report any instrument which becomes dangerously thin to the dentist. If this is not done then the tip could fracture during use and cause damage in the patients' mouth.

Scissors
Scissors, particularly suture scissors, become blunt after relatively few decontamination and sterilisation cycles. It is essential that suture scissors cut along their full length. In fact it is possibly more important that the tip is sharp, even if the rest of the blade is not so sharp, as it is usually only the tip is used to cut the suture. It is also important that the tips do not become bent and that they meet effectively.

It is possible to purchase sterile disposable suture scissors at less than the cost of their reusable equivalent. There are considerations about disposal of these scissors which will be covered in a subsequent chapter, but the fact that whenever needed they are guaranteed to be sharp could be worthy of serious consideration.

Crown shears may also need sharpening, but very infrequently and are difficult to sharpen because of their curved design.

Luxators and other elevators
The design and recommended use of luxators means that they need to be sharp to carry out their function effectively. Their principal function is to improve access for forceps when extracting teeth therefore they need to be sharp to perform this. Specific instructions for their care are included in the pack when bought as a set. The set also contains a flat and circular sharpening stone.

Extraction Forceps, Artery Forceps, Needle Holders and other Hinged Instruments
Any instrument that has a hinge or ratchets must be regularly checked for stiffness. The hinges of extraction forceps may need lubrication to ensure they work effectively.

Artery forceps, needle holders and other instruments with ratchets must be checked to ensure the ratchet works effectively and that the tips meet and are locked. If allowed to become slack they will not hold tissue or suture needles properly.

Tweezers

Tweezers, of whatever design, must have tips that meet properly. This also applies to tissue forceps used in surgical procedures. If the tips do not meet properly they will not hold the item being picked up. It is possible to buy locking tweezers that have plastic, replaceable locks. When metal locks are in place, care must be taken not to bend the locking arm, stopping it from engaging properly.

Orthodontic Pliers

Orthodontic pliers are very expensive instruments and need to be looked after to ensure a long usable life. They are specific to the task they perform therefore they must be kept in good order so that they perform their tasks effectively. Any maintenance advice given when bought must be followed.

The most important maintenance to be carried out on pliers is the lubrication of the joint. After use, the pliers should be decontaminated in an ultrasonic bath, if advised by the manufacturer, or manually cleaned, followed by lubrication using a recommended lubricant before sterilisation. They may need sterilisation at a lower temperature than other instruments and in a vacuum autoclave. This will be covered in more detail in a later chapter.

Sharpening Hand Instruments

The sharpening of scaling instruments forms an important component in the undergraduate teaching of dental and hygiene and therapy students in all courses held throughout the country. It is good practice to maintain sharp instruments for both the operator and the patient for the following reasons (University of Birmingham, 2006):

- Sharp instruments decrease operator fatigue as less force is required
- It decreases operator time as fewer strokes are required
- It increases precision as there is greater control over the instrument
- It reduces the burnishing of calculus
- It prevents trauma to the gingival tissues and therefore causes less patient discomfort
- It improves tactile sensitivity as a lighter grip is possible.

Goals to be achieved by sharpening:

- To produce a sharp edge
- To preserve the original instrument design
- To conserve the blades.

Sharpening dental instruments requires:

- Knowledge of the instrument design
- Skill
- Patience.

When does an instrument need sharpening?

The cutting edge is a fine line formed when the face and lateral surface meet at an angle. The edge therefore has length but not width. The edge becomes rounded during use and therefore has thickness and is dull (*Figure 1*). The aim of sharpening is to reshape the cutting edge to a fine line (*Figure 2*).

If checking visually, either with the naked eye or using loupes (10 times magnification): if the cutting edge is blunt it will be rounded, smooth and shiny and light will reflect from it. A dull non reflective line indicates sharpness.

The sharpness can also be checked by using an acrylic test stick. Test the cutting edge by applying it to the test stick as if on a tooth and draw it from heel to toe of the instrument.

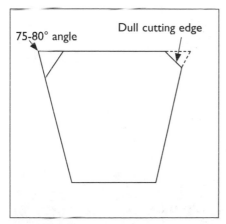

Figure 1. Shows how an edge dulls during use.

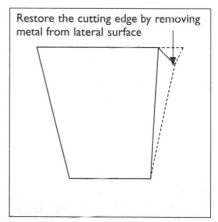

Figure 2. Restoration of a cutting edge. by removing metal from the lateral surface, shown by an arrow.

Manual Sharpening

This is carried out using a sharpening stone, which can be a natural stone (Arkansas is the usual stone used), or an artificial material such as a ceramic (*Figure 3*) and a lubricant, which can be oil or water. The manual sharpening process is:

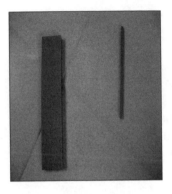

- Apply lubricant to stone and hold it on either side
- Check the angle and surface to be sharpened
- Rub the stone along the appropriate surface (*Figures 4,5,6* and *7*).
- If sharpening a probe, ensure that the whole circumference is sharpened.
- After sharpening is completed, sterilise the stone and the instrument.

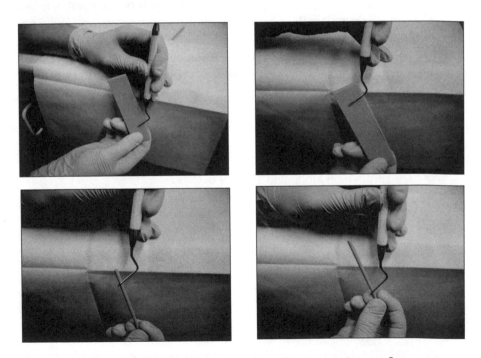

Figures 4, 5, 6, and 7. Rubbing the stone along the appropriate surface.

Apply only gentle pressure. Apply slightly more pressure on the downward stroke to prevent swarf — the tiny particles of metal — forming and building up against the sharpening surface. This stops the cutting edge actually contacting the stone surface and prevents effective sharpening. The tiny particles can also be picked up or blown into eyes or inhaled. Always finish on a downward stroke. The action of sharpening actually removes some of the metal of the instrument and the instrument must be very carefully checked as to whether the sharpened edge has made the instrument dangerously thin and liable to fracture during use.

After sharpening, even if the instrument was previously sterile, it must be sterilised again. It is advisable to decontaminate and sterilise an instrument before sharpening to avoid any risk of a needle stick injury. Manual sharpening can be used during treatment if an instrument becomes blunt because it is possible to sterilise the stone.

However, manual sharpening is very time consuming and requires very careful training to achieve a good result without damaging the instrument.

Mechanical Sharpening

There are many types of mechanical sharpening stone (*Figure 8*). The type featured in the following photographs is not the only type available and care should be taken to purchase the correct type for the purpose you require it for.

Mechanical sharpening stones work by electricity, so should be used with care. There is no need for a lubricant to be used but if used the sharpening is more efficient. Care must be taken not to sharpen for too long. It is also very easy to sharpen the wrong surface or at the wrong angle. Specific training is required and refreshers taken to ensure correct use. Only sterile instruments can be sharpened on an electric stone as the stone cannot be sterilised. The process is explained below:

- Ensure which angle and surface is to be sharpened
- Put correct surface at the required angle against the stone (*Figure 9*)
- Operate foot control to control the stone
- Check sharpness against test stick on side of wheel (*Figure 10*)
- Check to ensure the tip has not become dangerously thin
- Sterilise the instrument.

Instruments can become blunt by being bundled together and rubbing against each other during decontamination, sterilisation or storage.

It is possible for instruments to become pitted and rusty after years of use and decisions may have to be made as to their fitness for use. Companies that run Hospital Sterilisation and Decontamination Units (HSDUs) will examine

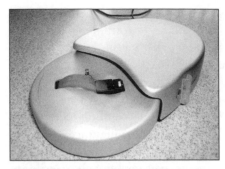

Figure 8. Example of an
electric sharpening stone.

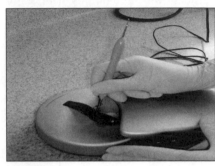

Figure 9. Sharpening a
curette.

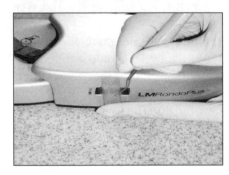

Figure 10. Checking sharpness
against an acrylic bar.

instruments and if they consider them to be a risk they will not process them.
This will include some instruments that have been engraved with a practice
name or number for example, or have coloured recognition tape on them as
they cannot ensure effective sterilisation of these areas.

Hand Pieces and other Rotary or Air Driven Instruments

Hand pieces are expensive, complicated instruments and require careful
maintenance and care. Different manufacturers have differing maintenance
and care recommendations. These instructions must be followed to the letter,
as failure to do so will result in breakdown and cause severe inconvenience
to the dental team. Maintenance contracts should be set up with approved

and certificated technicians. These handpieces cannot be serviced and maintained by the dentist or their staff.

Everyday maintenance and care is limited to cleaning, lubrication and sterilisation. The outside casing should be cleaned by wiping over with either an alcohol wipe or a disinfectant soaked cloth, before oiling, to remove any debris, blood and saliva. They should never be completely immersed in water or cleaned in an ultrasonic bath. This will remove all the lubrication from the intricate internal components, which cannot be effectively replaced.

Where a washer/disinfector is used before sterilisation, special racks can be bought to hold handpieces to ensure the internal lumens are effectively decontaminated. There are special decontamination, oiling and sterilising machines available on the market, specifically for handpieces.

Care should be taken when autoclaving handpieces, as not all components are autoclavable. Where they are all components must be oiled separately before or after autoclaving, depending on the manufacturer's advice. The same is true of sonic scalers, airscalers, cavitron handpieces and tips and any other rotary instruments.

Wherever possible handpieces and all other equipment which contain lumens, internal water pathways, should be sterilised in vacuum autoclaves as this is the only way to sterilise the lumen. This will be fully explained in a later chapter.

Electric micromotors are not usually autoclavable therefore careful decontamination must be carried out between patients and at the end of the session. They should be decontaminated to the manufacturer's instructions, using disinfectant solutions or alcohol wipes.

The water lines for handpieces must be run through without the handpieces attached at the start of the day for two minutes to help disperse any bacterial build up, and run through for about 20 or 30 seconds between patients to eliminate any bacteria in the lines. This is due to the back syphonage of contaminated water when the handpiece is stopped. It is recommended that bottled water systems are used whenever possible.

Suction Equipment

Most high speed evacuation is connected to the main waste dispersal from the unit and goes into the sewers. For this reason any local regulations must be adhered to and advice sought from the local water/sewerage service provider.

To keep the suction equipment working effectively any filters must be cleaned regularly, preferably daily, and a disinfectant solution run through the tubings. The unit manufacturer will advise on the correct solution to use. This solution is usually aspirated through the tubings using some form of container that also includes air in the aspiration. This will cause the solution to run round the inside surface of the tubing instead of just going straight down the centre, thus disinfecting the tubing more efficiently. This should be carried out at the end of the day at least if not at the end of every session.

The suction tubing should also have some water aspirated through it after every patient to help stop the build-up of mucous in the tubing.

Some new units have a built-in system to disinfect all the water lines and suction tubings. Again, the manufacturer's advice should be sought and instructions followed.

The use of mobile suction units is not advised as they are extremely difficult to decontaminate effectively and run a very real risk of significant bacterial build-up inside the apparatus — few of them have filters and the disposal of the bottle contents is difficult.

Electrical Equipment

The most important piece of electrical equipment is the dental unit. If this is not maintained well and cared for methodically then it causes considerable inconvenience to the dental team.

The unit must be subject to a maintenance contract and regular servicing. There is little that practice staff can do other than routine decontamination and cleaning, which must be carried out to the manufacturer's instructions. Nurses should never be expected to carry out maintenance, other than routine cleaning and disinfection. The only item that can be replaced is the light bulb and this should be undertaken by the dentist.

The other major piece of equipment that requires maintenance by specialist technicians, and never by practice staff, is the radiography equipment. There are legal requirements to ensure the safety of radiographic equipment (DH, 1999, 2000) as well as the safety of the users and the patients. The only maintenance that can be carried out by dental professionals is its basic cleaning and decontamination. Routine changing of the chemicals is carried out by practice staff, and no other maintenance should be undertaken by practice staff but by trained technicians on a contractual basis. The chemicals need to be changed regularly, depending on the number of radiographs being processed. If they are not changed regularly they will lose their effectiveness and radiographs will not be processed to an acceptable standard. The tanks inside the machine must be emptied, cleaned and refilled with new chemicals to maintain the quality of radiographic processing. The disposal of the spent chemicals is closely regulated and will be dealt with in a later chapter.

It is the responsibility of the dentist to ensure that all staff are trained in the use of equipment and this training is kept up to date and is logged. Any new equipment installed will need to be explained to staff and training given. The range of accessory electrical equipment, which is required in all dental surgeries, is vast and is being added to almost daily. It includes:

- Light curing lights
- Electric vitality testers
- Apex locators
- Cavitrons
- Endodontic ultrasonic motors
- Endodontic gutta percha heaters
- Endodontic heated gutta pluggers
- Electronic local anaesthetic delivery systems
- Inhalation sedation delivery systems
- Pulse oxymeters
- Blood pressure monitors
- Defibrillators
- Amalgamators/capsule mixers
- Electronic impression material mixing systems
- Dental lasers
- Radiography processing equipment
- Ceramic onlay makers
- Computer equipment
- Radiography viewers
- Laboratory equipment such as porcelain ovens
- Autoclaves
- Ultrasonic cleaners
- Washer/disinfectors.

This list is by no means exhaustive but is indicative of the diverse nature of accessory equipment required in the modern dental practice. The list will continue to grow as dentistry evolves and the technology becomes more advanced. The basic advice for the care and maintenance of all this type of equipment is, again, to 'follow the manufacturer's advice and instructions'. It is advisable to have spare batteries available as many of the smaller pieces of equipment are battery powered. Also make sure you have to hand electric vitality testers, apex locators, etc. Staff should also be conversant with the procedure for changing the batteries, i.e. how to gain access to the battery holder as it is not always as simple as it would appear.

Some of the auxiliary electrical equipment will have accessory items which will require care and maintenance. For example:

- Light curing lights have removable, autoclavable tips, which must be decontaminated carefully to remove any residual composite or bond before to autoclaving. Failure to do so can lead to insufficient light reaching the materials and ineffective curing

- Electric vitality testers will have removable tips, which will need to be decontaminated and sterilised after use and the machine itself will require wiping with alcohol or disinfectant
- Apex locators have lip clips and file holders, both of which require decontamination and sterilisation, with the machine again being wiped
- Cavitrons have removable autoclavable handles and tips. The reservoir must be emptied and the machine wiped after use
- Endodontic ultrasonic machines have handpieces and tips that are usually autoclavable, and they also have reservoirs that must be emptied. The needles on obturation machines are designated as single use and must only be used once, however expensive.

Most other accessory equipment is treated in the same way, i.e. wiped down after use with alcohol or disinfectant, but must never be allowed to become too wet as this could cause damage to the electrical circuits inside the machine. Other auxiliary equipment may be autoclavable or single use — check the product information.

Laboratory equipment must be maintained and subject to regular care again following the products' information. It is subject to the same regulations as dental instruments and requires a 'CE' mark to prove its acceptability. Some equipment can cause harm if not used and maintained correctly and training of new staff is as important in the laboratory as it is in the dental surgery. The laboratory manager will have the same responsibilities under law as the dental practice owner.

The efficient and effective care and maintenance of the equipment in a dental surgery or laboratory is essential to the smooth functioning of both. It is therefore essential that all new staff are trained in the correct use of equipment and when new items are purchased, are given appropriate training.

It is part of the 'duty of care' under the Health and Safety at Work Act 1974. It should also be remembered that all staff have the same duty of care and responsibility, under the same Act, which precludes them from performing any action which may put others or themselves at risk. This would include attempting inappropriate maintenance on dental equipment.

Dental nurses should be conversant with the correct working of equipment and be alert to malfunction of any kind in any appliance. They should bring this to the attention of the dentist or other person responsible for maintenance contracts at the earliest possible opportunity so that repairs can be carried out as soon as possible.

References

DH (1998) *Letter EL(98)5 – NHS Executive – January 1998.* Department of Health, London

DH (1999) *Ionising Radiation Regulations 1999 and subsequent amendments 2000.* HMSO, London

DH (2000) *Ionising Radiation (Medical Exposure) Regulations 2000.* HMSO, London

DH (1978) *Health und Safety at Work Act 1974.* HMSO, London

MHRA (1993) *Medical Devices Directive (93/42/EEC).* Medicines and Healthcare Products Regulatory Agency, London

MHRA (1994) *Medical Devices Regulations (SI 1994 No 3017).* Medicines and Healthcare Products Regulatory Agency (MHRA), London

MHRA (2002) *Medical Devices Regulations 2002.* Medicines and Healthcare Products Regulatory Agency, London

University of Birmingham (2006) *Sharpening of Scaling Instruments.* University of Birmingham School of Dentistry

CHECKLIST 4

Instruments are medical devices

- Medical Devices – definition.
- Medical Devices Regulations.
- Considerations to be taken when purchasing new equipment.
- Are there any waste disposal implications with the new equipment?

Care and Maintenance

- Mouth Mirrors
- Probes
- Excavators
- Carvers, Chisels and Cervical margin Trimmers
- Hand Scalers
- Luxators and elevators
- Extraction Forceps, Artery Forceps and other hinged instruments
- Tweezers
- Orthodontic pliers

Sharpening Hand Instruments

- Reasons for sharpening
- Goals to be achieved
- Requirements
- When to sharpen
- Manual sharpening – Arkansas and acrylic sharpening stones
- Mechanical sharpening stones

Handpieces and other rotary or air driven instruments

- Oiling
- Wiping not immersing in water or in ultrasonic baths.
- Specialist oiling, decontamination and sterilising machines
- Use vacuum autoclaves

Suction Equipment

- Cleaning filters
- Between patient aspiration of water
- Flushing with disinfectant
- Inadvisability of mobile units
- Electrical equipment
- Dental Chair and Unit
- Radiographic equipment.
- Accessory electrical equipment
- Auxiliary equipment care

Training in the use of new equipment

Duty of care under Health and Safety at work Act

Medicines and Healthcare Products Regulatory Agency advice.

CHAPTER 5

Decontamination and Sterilisation

The whole point of infection control is the removal of any risk of cross-contamination from one patient or person to another. Standard Precautions give us the basic requirements for this, and decontamination and sterilisation is a fundamental part of standard precautions.

There is little point in having effective hand washing, personal protective clothing, good cleaning regimes and effective care and maintenance of equipment if the pathogens left on the equipment by the treatment of one patient are still there when the next patient is treated — if the instrument is not effectively decontaminated and then sterilised there will be no infection control. Effective decontamination and sterilisation are fundamental to the whole infection control process.

Definitions

Cleaning
A process that removes contaminants including dust, soil (dirt), large numbers of micro-organisms and the organic matter, e.g. blood. Cleaning is an essential prerequisite to disinfection and sterilisation.

Disinfection
A process used to reduce the number of micro-organisms, but which does not usually kill or remove all micro-organisms rather it reduces them to a level which is not harmful to health.

Decontamination
A term used for the destruction or removal of microbial contamination to render an item safer to handle.

Antisepsis
A term meaning the prevention of sepsis or decay by killing or inhibiting micro-organisms. Now generally used for the treatment of skin, mucous membrane or other tissues.

Sanitisation

A process which reduces the number of microbes to an acceptable level.

Sterilisation

A process used to render an object free from all living organisms. It will not destroy prions.

For dental instruments contaminated during dental treatment the process of choice must be sterilisation unless the instrument has specific instructions from the manufacturer which call for disinfection or 'cold sterilisation'. Instruments treated in this way cannot be classified as sterile and must not be put with sterile instruments.

As described in the preceding definitions, cleaning is an essential prerequisite of decontamination and sterilisation. It is the basis for maintenance of large pieces of equipment before disinfection.

Disinfection is carried out on surfaces or items that cannot be sterilised, using agents usually recommended by the manufacturer.

Decontamination is an essential prerequisite of sterilisation. It is not sufficient for instruments contaminated during dental treatment to be simply decontaminated and reused.

Sterilisation is the only way to ensure that all micro-organisms and pathogens have been killed and cannot be transmitted to another patient. However, sterilisation will not destroy prions as they are not living organisms.

Legal Matters

The decontamination and sterilisation of medical devices is the subject of a large number of Acts of Parliament, Health Technical Memoranda (HTM) and European Commission Regulations. Although there is no specific 'Decontamination and Sterilisation Act' as such, there are many aspects that are covered within Health and Safety Legislation (see *Appendix 1* at the end of this chapter). The overriding document which gives comprehensive information, rules and regulations and sets the standards for all aspects of decontamination and sterilisation is Health Technical Memorandum 01-01 (DH, 2007). This document seeks to bring together earlier Health Technical Memoranda.

Other significant documents include *Protocol for the Local Decontamination of Reusable Medical Devices* (DH, 2001) and *A Guide to the Decontamination of reusable Surgical Instruments* (DH, 2003). Both of these documents are long and very detailed but they provide the basis for agreed procedures and policies drawn up by NHS Trusts. The British Dental Association (BDA, 2003) gives a sample infection control policy and this should form the basis of general dental practice infection control policies.

All personnel who undertake cleaning, decontamination and sterilisation are subject to the *Personal Protective Equipment Regulations* (DH, 1992), the *Reporting of Injuries, Diseases and Dangerous Occurrences Regulations* (RIDDOR) (DH, 1995) and the Health and Safety at Work Act 1974.

Instruments are subject to the Medical Devices Directive (MHRA, 1993) and the Medical Devices Regulations (MHRA, 1994). The equipment required for decontamination and sterilisation is subject to legislation. This includes the Pressure Systems Regulations 1989 (Health and Safety Executive [HSE], 1989), and the Pressure Systems Safety Regulations 2001 (HSE, 2000) and Health Technical Memoranda (see *Appendix 1*). The Health and Safety Executive also publishes an approved code of practice (ACOP) *Safety of Pressure Systems*. This equipment is also subject to the Medical devices Regulations and Directives.

The dentist has a duty of care under the Health and Safety at Work act 1974 as well as a responsibility to ensure that all decontamination and sterilisation equipment complies with the Medical Devices Directives and Regulations. They must provide training in the correct use of the equipment. They must provide appropriate personal protective equipment and if an accident should happen, report it to the appropriate authority under RIDDOR guidance.

The dentist should also have some knowledge of the protocol for the decontamination of medical devices and for surgical instruments.

The dental nurse has to perform the practical cleaning, decontamination and sterilisation of the instruments and equipment but must be appropriately trained to perform these tasks competently and safely. The nurse must be prepared to ask for training or explanations of their expectations and be prepared to undertake training.

A trained, qualified nurse will have received all the background knowledge required as well as a basic training in the use of the equipment. It should be remembered, however, that equipment varies greatly and when entering a new work environment the nurse may require training in the specific use of the equipment installed and used.

The NHS Estates Decontamination Project (DH, 2001) sets out minimum requirements for NHS establishments and the use of central sterilisation facilities. These facilities are purpose built to decontaminate and sterilise large numbers of instruments and pieces of equipment from many sources in optimum conditions to the highest possible standards. Contracts are set up and systems evolved for the collection of contaminated items, transport to the facility for reprocessing, and the return of sterile instruments. These facilities are registered and their processes validated before commencement of reprocessing.

Track and Trace

Instruments and equipment sterilised in these facilities are subject to 'Track and Trace'. This is the ability to track and trace instruments and equipment through the decontamination life cycle and enables corrective action to be taken when necessary, i.e. in the unlikely event of a sterilisation cycle failure products can then be recalled.

Track and Trace is usually accomplished by using a series of bar coded labels affixed to the item and a tag which stays with it, inside its covering, during processing. The outer label is scanned and the tray or instrument used. After use the tray or instrument will be scanned again before being sent for reprocessing. The item will be scanned again on receipt at the facility and throughout the decontamination and sterilisation process. This process requires the installation of computers with specific software to record the scanning.

The records held in the computer are not only used to trace an item in the event of a recall, but also for audit purposes. The track and trace system tracks the instrument through all the decontamination and sterilisation process, right through to the patient and then back again. It is unrealistic to expect individual dental practices to have such systems, but the NHS Decontamination Project (DH, 2001) seeks to bring dental practices as well as chiropody clinics and other ancillary health professionals into the system to standardise decontamination and sterilisation across the whole healthcare spectrum.

The Decontamination Life Cycle

The whole cycle from purchase of an item of equipment, through its use, decontamination, sterilisation and ultimate destruction is illustrated in *Figure 1*. It is essential that set standards are achieved at every stage of the cycle, from purchase to destruction. If the agreed standards are not met at any stage then the final result will be ineffective decontamination and possible cross contamination. There are certain issues which must be addressed at each stage of the cycle:

- The location where the decontamination takes place
- The facilities and equipment at the location
- The equipment used is validated, maintained and tested in accordance with manufacturer's instructions and legislation
- There are effective management systems in place to ensure policies and procedures are followed
- Policies and procedures for all aspects of the process are agreed, implemented and monitored.

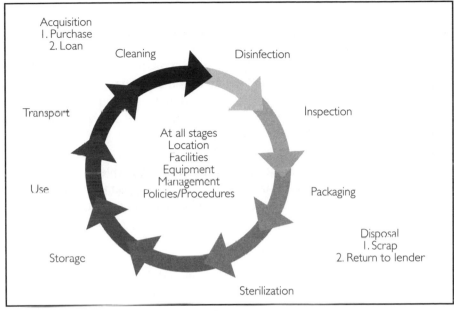

Figure 1: The Decontamination life cycle.

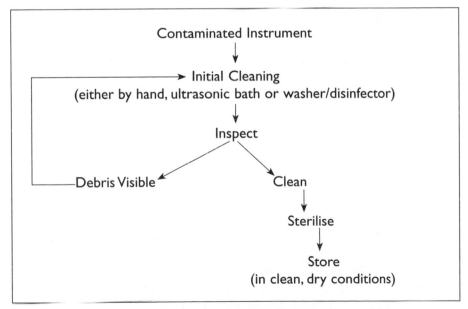

Figure 2. Decontamination flow chart (British Dental Association, 2003).

In 2002 the Department of Health published standards for the decontamination of reusable medical devices (DH, 2002), against which all healthcare facilities and establishments are audited. All facilities and establishments should meet these standards and are all subject to regular audit, after which action plans are drawn up to address any shortcomings and are agreed between the auditor and the facility management.

It is, again, unrealistic for general dental practitioners to have decontamination systems which are as comprehensive as those which are purpose-built, industrial-sized facilities, but the basic and fundamental decontamination cycle must be followed and high standards must be maintained. The BDA (2003) has a flow diagram which gives a simple guide to the decontamination process and is a good reference point (see *Figure 2*).

When setting up a decontamination area in whatever sized establishment, it should contain the following:

- Separate 'clean' and 'dirty' areas
- Facilities in the 'dirty' area to clean and decontaminate, contaminated instruments and equipment
- Facilities in the 'clean' area to sterilise the decontaminated equipment
- Storage arrangements for the clean, dry, safe storage of the sterilised equipment.

The 'Dirty' Area

The 'dirty' or decontamination area should contain a designated decontamination sink. If there is no mechanical means of decontamination, then this sink must be deep enough to allow the contaminated items to be completely immersed in water in the sink. If there is other decontamination equipment available, i.e. an ultrasonic cleaner or a washer/disinfector, then this sink need not be so deep. However it should be of an adequate size and depth to allow instruments to be rinsed before mechanical decontamination and again after decontamination.

Sink
This area should also contain a designated hand-wash sink which does not have a plug so that hand washing is only carried out under running water and no decontamination can be carried out This should be fitted with appropriate soap dispenser and paper towels. Staff must be able to wash their hands after removing rubber gloves used during instrument decontamination and before leaving the area.

Lubricating handpieces

There should also be facilities to clean and lubricate handpieces and their component parts. This could consist of cans of oil with appropriate nozzles to facilitate effective lubrication, or an oiling machine which gives a measured dose of oil. If handpieces are lubricated before sterilisation then it should be carried out in the decontamination room. However, if lubrication is carried out after sterilisation to follow manufacturer's instructions, then the handpieces should be wiped over to remove debris in the dirty area and then taken to the clean area to be sterilised. The lubrication equipment must be kept in the clean area and not transferred. This may entail the purchase of two sets of lubrication equipment if some items are lubricated before sterilisation and some after as the same equipment cannot be used for both.

Storage and disposal bin

The decontamination area should also contain storage space for cleaning materials and solvents for the mechanical decontamination machines. There must be heavy-duty rubber gloves, protective glasses, masks and disposable plastic aprons available. There should also be a clinical waste bin with appropriate bags. This bin should be foot operated and have a close fitting lid.

The 'dirty' area should also have the facilities and solutions for the disinfection of non-sterilisable items and for the decontamination of impressions before sending to the laboratory, and the disinfection of any items that need to be sent for repair.

Preparation of solutions

This area should be used for the preparation of solutions for the decontamination of the dental unit, chair and other accessory equipment before, during and after the treatment session, and it would be good practice to have available written procedure sheets for the making-up of solutions and advice on immediate action to be taken in the event of any solution or contaminated water being splashed into the eyes or ingestion of any of the chemicals. Chemicals stored in this area should be stored safely, with lids tightly screwed on. Any containers used to disinfect items that cannot be sterilised must have close fitting lids, which should be in place at all times. Good ventilation in this area will help to disperse any fumes from chemicals used. Solutions made up at the start of the day must be disposed of at the end of the day and new solutions made up next day.

Disinfection

Items which can only be disinfected should be processed in the 'dirty' area and not allowed to contaminate the 'clean' area. Disinfection does not render the item pathogen-free — it only reduces the microbial load and cannot ensure the complete eradication of all microbes. Disinfection must never be used as an alternative to sterilisation to 'save time'.

Items which can only be disinfected include:

- Protective glasses or goggles
- Reusable plastic bibs
- Surfaces of equipment
- Air syringe handles
- Exposed handpiece tubing
- Suction tubing
- Some photographic mirrors
- Some cheek retractors.

There are many disinfectants available and the manufacturers of the equipment will recommend which is appropriate for their product. This advice should be followed at all times. The disinfectant used should have a virucidal, bactericidal and fungicidal action. Check the name of the product that you are using:

-cidal means 'kills micro-organisms'
-static means 'inhibits growth and reproduction'

Therefore check that the solution to be used is *–cidal,* not *–static*, to ensure it will kill as many pathogens as possible.

Care should be taken to check any relevant Control of Substances Hazardous to Health regulations (DH, 1998) relating to the disinfectants used. They should always be used to recommended solution strengths and not diluted more than recommended as this will reduce the effectiveness. Some disinfectants emit harmful fumes so good ventilation is required.

Disinfectant solutions must be made up daily and disposed of, safely, at the end of the day. Containers used should be clearly labelled with the name and strength of the solution. The containers of concentrated solutions, or tablets which some solutions are supplied as, must be stored safely and to the manufacturer's instructions. They should never be stored in an area which is accessible to the general public. When choosing a disinfectant consider:

- Can the item be sterilised — this must be the process of choice if compatible with the instruments' manufacture.
- If sterilisation is impossible, then the disinfectant:
    - Should have a wide range of microbial activity
    - If used for surfaces, it should have a rapid, disinfection, action

- Should not be easily neutralised by organic matter, soaps, hard water or plastics
- Should be non-corrosive at optimum concentration
- Should be non-irritant if used for skin disinfection
- Should be inexpensive
- Should not emit harmful fumes.

The 'Clean' Area

The 'clean' area should, ideally, be totally separate from the 'dirty' area but easily accessible from the 'dirty' area. It is a health and safety and manual handling risk to carry decontaminated but unsterile equipment around from one area to another. This is impractical in small dental practices. As long as a strict regime of glove changing and hand washing is in place and complied with, then the two areas can be adjacent. There must be, however a strict barrier between the two and no temptation to 'borrow' from one area to the other.

The Autoclave

The 'clean' area should contain the means of sterilising the decontaminated equipment, i.e. the autoclave. There are two types of autoclave: the displacement autoclave and the vacuum phase autoclave. The differences between them and their differing uses will be explained later in the chapter.

Autoclaves which have a vacuum phase or drying cycle can sterilise instruments in pouches as the vacuum or drying cycle will ensure the instruments come out dry. Such packets should be sealed with autoclave tape which contains chemical stripes which change colour when the optimum sterilising conditions are reached. Such instruments are sterile until the packet is opened or inadvertently punctured.

Autoclaves that do not have such a cycle will leave the instruments wet at the end of the cycle. These instruments must be carefully dried, ideally using sterile paper towels and then bagged in instrument pouches. Some will argue that bagging is not necessary, but this will ensure that instruments cannot become contaminated from environmental contamination before use. Such instruments should be bagged as soon as they are taken from the autoclave and after being dried. These instruments are not 'sterile' but have been 'sterilised'. As soon as they are taken out of the autoclave and come into contact with the air they are no longer sterile.

There should be a designated clean area alongside the autoclave to receive sterilised items. Ideally this area will have a sterile disposable cover. There should also be storage space for chemical indicators and testing log books and the pyrogen — free water for refilling the autoclaves.

The packs should be treated in the same way as sterile packs, in so much as they are clean until opened or inadvertently punctured. Although not 'sterile' they should be considered as contaminated by environmental contamination, and if the packet is punctured the instrument should be reprocessed.

If all sterilised instruments are stored in the surgery care must be taken not to contaminate the packets when taking other packets from storage. Strict glove and hand hygiene must be adhered to. Infrequently used equipment or instruments can be stored in the 'clean' area in suitable clean and dry cupboards.

With careful and thorough training, robust policies and procedures and strict monitoring in place it is possible for a general dental practice to achieve and maintain a high standard of decontamination and sterilisation. The trained and efficient dental nurse will want to ensure that these high standards are upheld by having those same high standards themselves and by not allowing others to make do with anything less. Should other, specially employed personnel undertake this essential function, then rigorous training and monitoring is essential.

In basic terms, the arrangement of the clean and dirty areas in a dental practice is not fundamentally different from those in a purpose-built facility. The same high standard can be achieved even if there is no separate decontamination room but just a decontamination area set aside in the main surgery; with careful planning and strict adherence to good practice acceptable decontamination and sterilisation can be achieved.

It is an almost impossible task to expect a dental nurse to work at the chairside and carry out effective decontamination and sterilisation all in the same area without there being some accidental contamination of sterilised items about to be used or just been sterilised.

The Decontamination Process

To achieve effective decontamination and sterilisation of reusable medical devices, the requirements of all the Medical Devices Directives and Regulations must be fulfilled. This should be checked before purchase and consideration of these requirements should be part of the process undertaken before purchase of the equipment — whether it is the smallest hand instrument or the largest dental chair and unit. This is presumed to have been complied with before the decontamination life cycle starts.

Cleaning

This must be carried out on even brand new, just-out-of-the-packet instruments and is the essential pre-requisite to decontamination and sterilisation.

Process: Manual cleaning — by washing — is a soil (debris) removing process which requires energy and which results in the physical removal of a proportion of micro-organisms without achieving microbial destruction. Only use manual methods when other mechanical methods are inappropriate or unavailable.

Preferred uses: Decontaminating the surgery environment (floors, walls, furniture and fittings and equipment).

Exclusions: Cleaning is not acceptable for final decontamination for invasive equipment in direct contact with the patient, for which disinfection and sterilisation is required. It is also not acceptable on items designated as 'single use'.

Equipment required:
- Immersion method: A sink deep enough to hold sufficient water/detergent to totally immerse the items to be cleaned.
- Wiping method: Receptacle to hold water/detergent solution and disposable cloths.
- In addition, for both methods, a sink for rinsing and paper towels for drying.

Factors influencing effectiveness:
- Water temperature
- Concentration of detergent solution
- Nature and method of soil (dirt) removal
- Nature of item being cleaned and how accessible it is for cleaning of all surfaces.

Risks involved: Water logging of electrical equipment.

Safety: Personal protective clothing must be worn when cleaning fixtures and fittings, heavy duty rubber gloves, glasses and a disposable apron. Examination gloves are not suitable for use when cleaning.

Disinfection

There is a distinct difference between disinfection and decontamination: Instruments for sterilisation are decontaminated; instruments which cannot be sterilised are disinfected.

Disinfection of non-sterilisable items
Some items of equipment are not able to be sterilised. This includes:

- Some cheek retractors
- Some photographic mirrors
- Protective glasses/goggles
- Plastic protective, reusable bibs for patients.

The smaller items can be 'cold sterilised', and although it is not as effective as sterilisation it can render the item 'suitable for reuse'. These items are not invasive items and should not be used in invasive procedures during treatment. Once the items are clean they are soaked in a suitable decontaminant (which will be recommended by the manufacturer). The decontaminants used should have bactericidal, virucidal and fungicidal actions. They can be the same as the solutions used to decontaminate items before laboratory transfer or before repair by outside technicians and must be diluted to the recommended solution strength. If this immersion method is used, the item must be totally immersed in the solution for the recommended length of time in a suitable container with a tight fitting lid. Personal protective clothing should be worn and care taken not to inhale any fumes from the solution. It is advised that a Control of Substances Hazardous to Health assessment is carried out for all decontaminants used. This assessment should be written and be kept up-to-date when solution types are changed. It should be readily available within the environment that the solution is used to facilitate prompt action in the event of an accident.

For larger items (including protective glasses) the only way to disinfect them is by wiping. They should be wiped after every use with either an alcohol solution — specially produced for this purpose — or with a disposable cloth with an approved decontaminant solution applied (which must then be thrown away). It is possible to purchase alcohol wipes in a tub for this type of use. These wipes are efficient but there is a danger of them drying out if the lid is not closed properly. If a bleach solution is used the item must be carefully dried before reuse so that the bleach is not carried onto the patient or users' clothing or face.

Single use items must never be disinfected for reuse.

Decontamination Before Sterilisation

There are two methods of decontamination before sterilisation:

- Manual
- Mechanical.

Manual Decontamination
Instruments and other sterilisable equipment which is to be manually

decontaminated has to be capable of withstanding total immersion in water, if this is not possible, then the item should be wiped over.

Immersible items should be placed in a designated sink. Instruments should not be decontaminated in the same sink as is used for hand-washing. The instruments should be totally immersed in a water/detergent solution and cleaned under the water. If a brush is used, it should be reserved for this process only and should, ideally, be autoclaved after every use or should be disposable and thrown away after every use.

After cleaning, the instruments should be closely examined to ensure all debris has been removed, then rinsed in clean water and dried using disposable paper towels, taking care to avoid inoculation injuries. They can then be loaded onto autoclave trays, ensuring there is space around each instrument, and loaded into the autoclave. This is essential to allow the steam to contact all surfaces of the instruments to ensure effective sterilisation.

Mechanical Decontamination
There are two main types of mechanical decontamination equipment in use:

- Washer/disinfectors
- Ultrasonic baths.

Washer/Disinfectors
Process: Washer/disinfectors use a combination of physical cleaning and thermal microbial action to achieve disinfection/decontamination of contaminated, sterilisable equipment. This process should be used before sterilisation, not instead of.

Preferred Uses: This process can only be used on equipment that will withstand wet heat at temperatures of 80°C on repeated occasions. They must be capable of withstanding powerful water jets and alkaline detergents. For items such as anaesthetic tubing and masks this process may be sufficient to allow reuse, but single use types or sterilisable would be preferred. For sterilisable equipment, this process should be used to remove gross contamination and make the equipment safer to handle.

Exclusions: Single use items must not be put through a washer/disinfector. Equipment with an internal lumen, unless special adaptors are fitted to allow hollow and lumen items to be satisfactorily decontaminated. This process does not sterilise the items and they must be sterilised after decontamination.

Equipment required: A purpose built, suitably sized, washer/disinfector. It should have a thermostatically linked cycle and safety systems built in to prevent opening during the cycle. It should have internal racks to accept trays of instruments which must allow water spray to reach all aspects. Suitable detergents and decontaminants and rinse aids are released during the cycle, from an automatic dispenser or reservoir. Water softeners may be required in some areas.

Operating procedure:
- A series of cool or warm water washes with detergent to remove soil (dirt) at below protein coagulation temperatures
- A series of rinses to remove residual detergent
- A phase or cycle that achieves a temperature of at least 71°C for 3 minutes, 80°C for at least 1 minute or 90°C for at least 1 second, in all parts of the load, usually the final rinse
- A heat-assisted drying cycle.

Monitoring: The machine must be commissioned with temperature measurements in a 'worst case' load so that the most inaccessible portions reach at least 71°C for at least 3 minutes. The chamber cycle parameters should be noted and rechecked routinely and monitoring should occur in such a way that any gross failure in water supply or electrical power results in clear indication of a failed cycle. It should not be possible to remove any load in the normal manner if this occurs. Cleaning efficiency should be monitored using a standard 'soil' test.

Maintenance: The washer/disinfector must be maintained to the manufacturer's instructions. Each load must be checked after washing to ensure effective cleaning. Routine thermometric checks must also be performed. Maintenance of the actual machinery must be carried out by a trained, accredited technician.

Advantages: This is a safe process for the operator. There is good disinfection of items by cleaning and heat, minimal handling of grossly contaminated items by staff, and it results in clean items.

Disadvantages: The equipment is initially expensive to buy and requires adequately trained staff to operate and load correctly. Planned preventative maintenance costs may be high and will include routine thermometric monitoring. It may require artificially softened water. The detergents used could be irritant to the skin of operators. The cycle can take 45 minutes or even longer to complete.

Area of action: The use of a washer/disinfector will inactivate all micro-organisms except bacterial spores and some heat resistant viruses. It does not destroy prions and may not remove them completely.

Safety precautions: Personal protective clothing must be used and care with handling the detergents. A COSHH assessment will need to be carried out.

Ultrasonic Baths

Process: These use high frequency sound waves which are radiated through the liquid medium. As the sound waves pass through the liquid, they cause the formation of tiny bubbles. As these bubbles grow in size they become unstable and implode. This causes the cleaning fluid to rush in and fill the gap. This action, repeated thousands of times every second in every cubic centimetre of the fluid, gives ultrasonic cleaners their powerful cleaning action and makes them the most effective method for the removal of debris and contaminants from hard surfaces and complex shapes. This action is aided by the addition of detergents or enzymatic solutions. Enzymatic solutions are particularly effective at removing mucus or saliva contaminated debris, as they help to break down the enzymes contained in the saliva, which add to its 'stickiness'.

Preferred uses: Equipment capable of withstanding total immersion in water. Should be used to remove gross contamination before sterilisation, and make equipment safer to handle.

Exclusions: Single use items must never be put through the ultrasonic bath. Air-driven handpieces and all their components should not be put through an ultrasonic bath. This process does not sterilise the items and they must be sterilised after cleaning/decontamination.

Equipment required: A purpose-built, suitably sized ultrasonic bath. It should have a timing device, a close-fitting lid and a drainage tube or tap. It must have a basket which hangs from the sides of the bath and does not touch the bottom of the bath. Suitable detergent/enzymatic solutions need to be diluted to the manufacturer's instructions.

Operating procedure:
- Close drain tube or tap and fill bath to advised level with water and a recommended enzymatic detergent
- Put dirty instruments into the basket and place in bath, having rinsed first to remove loose debris
- Put on close fitting lid
- Start bath and operate for the recommended time span
- Remove basket and rinse instruments under running water
- Check for visible cleanliness
- If visibly clean, dry and sterilise. If still contaminated repeat or manually clean.

Monitoring: The bath must never be turned on when empty of water. 'Soil' tests must be carried out regularly and the length of time taken to fully remove soil, used as the minimum cleaning time per load. Regular electrical testing to check efficiency of machine should be carried out by trained technicians and documented.

Maintenance: The bath should be drained when the solution becomes grossly contaminated and dirty. This may be at the end of the session, the end of the day or during a session, depending on use and amount of debris on instruments. It must be emptied at the end of the day, washed out and dried and left unplugged. Regular 'soil' tests should be carried out to check optimum cleaning times. Repair and maintenance of the machinery should be carried out by trained and qualified technicians.

Advantages: It is a safer process than manual cleaning, but less safe than washer/disinfectors. It renders the equipment clean in the majority of cases, and safer for staff to handle.

Disadvantages: The machines are relatively expensive and an appropriate size must be purchased. Training is required for safe use.

Area of action: Ultrasonic cleaning will inactivate microbes but not viruses or bacterial spores.

Safety precautions: Personal protective clothing must be worn. The bath must never be operated without a tight fitting lid. The bubbles produced during the process will burst on the surface and cause a contaminated aerosol. A COSHH assessment should be carried out for the detergent/ enzymatic solution used.

It must be stressed that the preceding processes only decontaminate the equipment processed. Unless specified by the manufacturer, the items must be sterilised after processing. These processes must never be used as an alternative to sterilisation.

Single use items must never be decontaminated for reuse: some need to be sterilised before use and then disposed of afterwards. This will be outlined in the manufacturer's instructions.

These processes should be completed in the 'dirty' area of the decontamination room. Once decontaminated, the instruments should be dried and prepared for sterilisation. They may or may not require bagging, depending on the type of autoclave used. It is at this stage that orthodontic pliers, forcep hinges and handpiece components should be lubricated (except in the cases where the manufacturer recommends lubrication after sterilisation).

After lubrication the items are placed on autoclave trays. The items should be spaced apart as the steam will not penetrate in between touching items. If a vacuum autoclave is being used, then the instruments can be placed in an appropriately sized pouch and sealed using autoclave indicator tape. This indicator tape will confirm that the correct temperature and pressure were attained, but is not a substitute for regular efficient monitoring of the autoclave. The tape will appear with brown stripes after sterilising if the correct sterilising conditions are reached. Pouches usually have an indicator on the paper side which fulfils the same purpose. Most pouches are see-through on one side and paper on the other.

Unsterilised trays of instruments should be kept in the 'dirty' area until space is available in the autoclave and should then be put straight from the 'dirty' area into the autoclave. The autoclave chamber should not be overfilled as this will prevent effective steam penetration and ineffective sterilisation.

Care must be taken when loading the autoclave not to contaminate any of the surfaces, door handles, etc. in the 'clean' area with dirty gloves.

Wrapping

After decontamination, visual checking and drying, instruments can be sterilised. If vacuum phase autoclaves are used then instruments can be wrapped in pouches, or trays of instruments can be wrapped in cloth wraps to facilitate aseptic opening (discussed in a later section).

There is a recommended way to seal autoclave pouches to enable users to open them without contaminating the contents and to ensure effective sterilisation. This is illustrated in *Figure 3*.

Pouches closed in this way should be opened by cutting the tape and unfolding the folded down top. The instruments should then be dropped out onto a clean surface ideally covered by a sterile cover. The instruments should never be pushed out through the paper side of the pouch as this could cause contamination.

There are two ways of folding wraps and covering trays of instruments, both of which allow aseptic opening: they are known as the 'parcel fold' (*Figure 4*) and the 'envelope fold' (*Figure 5*).

Both techniques follow a complex path of folds to prevent the entry of contamination or contaminants. They both allow aseptic opening to be carried out.

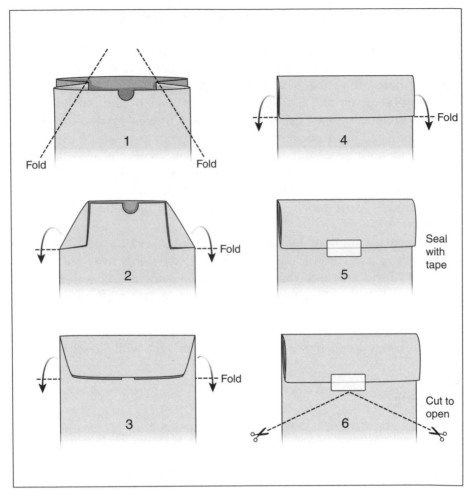

Figure 3. Aseptic closing for autoclave pouches.

Sterilisation

There are four main types of sterilising processes:

- Hot air sterilisation
- Chemical sterilisation
- Irradiation
- Steam sterilisation

Hot Air Sterilisation

This method of sterilisation uses high temperatures over long periods of time.

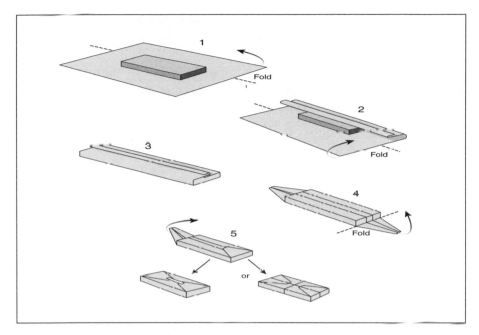

Figure 4. The parcel fold technique.

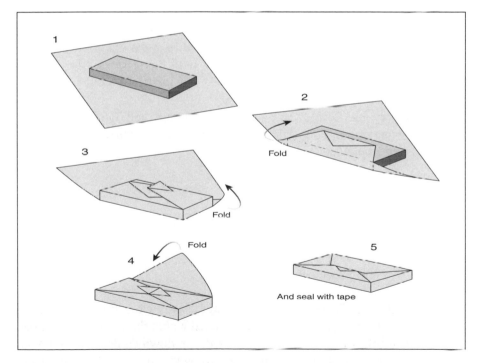

Figure 5. The envelope fold technique.

It was used in the past for some sensitive instruments and it was believed that sharp instruments were not blunted as quickly during hot air sterilisation as they are during steam or wet heat sterilisation.

However, more recent evidence has found that hot air sterilisation is not to be recommended for the sterilisation of reusable medical devices. When used the operating sterilisation was 160°C for two hours. This would be totally impractical for dental practices.

Chemical sterilisation

Delicate instruments and instruments that could not withstand either high temperatures or moisture, used to be sterilised by placing them in a closed container containing formaldehyde tablets. The formaldehyde emitted would sterilise the item in the container. This was ceased as a routine method of local sterilisation as instruments became more robust and able to withstand steam sterilisation. There was also an inherent risk from the formaldehyde fumes.

Chemical sterilisation is still carried out on industrial scales and is often used to sterilise disposable items. The chemical of choice is now ethylene oxide.

Irradiation

Irradiation sterilisation uses X-rays, Gamma rays and subatomic particles and cannot be undertaken in a dental practice. It is most commonly used to sterilise or irradiate food. There are dangers with the processes for each of these methods and they can only be carried out in strictly controlled areas with stringent safety procedures in place.

In dentistry, sterile gloves, gauze swabs, wraps and sterile gowns are sterilised using irradiation. All the processes are the subject of a British Standard (see *Appendix 1*).

Steam Sterilisation

There are two main types of benchtop steam steriliser:

- Displacement autoclaves
- Vacuum phase autoclaves.

Displacement autoclaves: Displacement autoclaves work by displacing the air in the autoclave by steam. Steam is produced within the autoclave chamber. The steam displaces the air, either upwards or downwards, depending on type. This displacement increases the pressure within the chamber. The steam condenses creating a wet load. Instruments sterilised in this way ideally need to be used straight away or dried, bagged and stored. Ideally they should be dried using sterile paper towels and then bagged in steriliser pouches and sealed. Instruments dried and bagged can be stored in dry conditions. Such instruments cannot be considered 'sterile' and only that 'they have been sterilised'. This situation is acceptable for routine dental instruments as long as the instruments are stored correctly and the autoclave has had all its mandatory checks, but it is not acceptable for surgical instruments. It is also imperative that the instruments are dried using sterile paper towels and bagged immediately as they are taken from the autoclave and not allowed to sit around in the open before bagging — they could not then be safely used as they could have been exposed to environmental contamination.

Displacement autoclaves cannot effectively sterilise the lumen inside handpieces, etc. or hollow instruments of any kind.

The cycle time for displacement autoclaves is shorter. The cycle starts by water, pyrogen-free, being taken from the reservoir into the chamber, where it is heated and steam produced. The pressure inside the chamber increases as the air is displaced. When the temperature and pressure reach a set level, for a sustained time, the sterilisation cycle begins. This cycle varies depending on the setting required and is activated when the autoclave is first started.

Most commonly used Autoclave cycles: The most common cycle used is 134°C holding temperature for a minimum of 3 minutes. The longer cycles at lower pressures are used for more delicate instruments and items such as photographic mirrors or cheek retractors. Care should be taken to ensure the correct cycle is used so that the instruments or items are not damaged (see *Table 1*). At the end of this time the steam condenses back into the reservoir. Once the chamber has completely decompressed the cycle is completed and the autoclave can be opened. There are warning lights at each stage and usually a visual display showing the temperature and pressure. The lights move across a panel as each phase is completed and eventually a light shows 'cycle complete'. It is at this time that the autoclave can be opened and emptied.

Throughout the cycle, once started, there are safety features built in to make it impossible for the autoclave to be opened. These take the form of

Table 1. Most commonly used autoclave cycles

Minimum Temperature	Maximum Temperature	Pressure (Bars)	Minimum Time
134°C	137°C	2.25	3 Minutes
126°C	129°C	1.50	10 Minutes
121°C	124°C	1.15	15 Minutes

bolts that fly across the door hinges and prevent the door from opening, and a pressure seal on the door. These features are some of the weekly checks which must be carried out on each autoclave. Should this mechanism fail and someone tried to open the door when the pressure has built up it would cause the autoclave door to be blown off and the person standing by it could sustain a severe or possibly even fatal injury.

Vacuum phase autoclaves: Vacuum autoclaves also sterilise by high temperature steam and the creation of a vacuum within the autoclave chamber. The vacuum is created at the start of the cycle and removes all moisture from the instruments, including the lumen and hollow parts, allowing the steam to contact all surfaces and producing a dry load. It is possible to purchase benchtop autoclaves with this feature for dental practices. The fact that the items are dry at the end of the cycle makes it possible to sterilise items in pouches. The items are sterile until the pouch is opened or inadvertently punctured. This is the recommended means of sterilising all instruments with lumen or hollow parts and for orthodontic pliers. For all these reasons, vacuum phase autoclaves should be the autoclave of choice when new machines are being purchased.

Vacuum phase autoclaves are much more complex and require more rigorous testing. They are also more expensive to buy and because of the 'drying' vacuum phase they take longer to sterilise items. The cycle sequence is similar to that of the displacement autoclave, with the addition of the vacuum phase at the end.

Care and Maintenance of Autoclaves

The care, maintenance and safe use of autoclaves is outlined documents summarised in *Appendix 1*. There are certain maintenance procedures which must be carried out daily, weekly, quarterly, and yearly. The BDA (2003) details the service and maintenance requirements. It stresses that all servicing and maintenance must be carried out, following the manufacturer's instructions.

Vacuum autoclaves require more rigorous testing and this should be taken into consideration when purchasing a new autoclave. A service and maintenance agreement should cover anticipated response times in the event of a breakdown.

- Autoclaves must be validated before use and their performance monitored routinely (by periodic testing, including daily and weekly user tests)
- The equipment must be properly maintained according to the manufacturer's instructions
- Correct operation of the autoclave must be checked whenever the

autoclave is used by recording the readings (physical parameters) on the autoclave's instruments or printout at the beginning of each clinical session
- The readings should be compared with the recommended values — if any reading is outside its specified limits, the sterilisation cycle must be regarded as unsatisfactory, irrespective of the results obtained from chemical indicators, and the autoclave cycle checked again. If the second cycle is unsatisfactory, the autoclave should not be used until the problem has been rectified by an engineer
- Autoclave logs and printouts should be retained for inspection and monitoring to demonstrate that the autoclave is performing within the recommended parameters.

At the end of each day the residual water should be drained from the autoclave chamber and reservoir, which should then be cleaned and left open to dry overnight. If no drainage facility is incorporated in the autoclave and one cannot be fitted, the high volume suction should be used, when the water has cooled, only if the autoclave is within reach. The autoclave should not be lifted or moved. The water used to refill the reservoir must be pyrogen free and not contain any minerals.

Newer autoclaves of both types can have printers fitted to give written proof of correct working. If there is no printout facility then the autoclave must be checked by watching the display during the cycle and the times are within agreed parameters. These checks must be recorded and kept for inspection in a designated log.

It is possible to chemically check the efficiency of the sterilisation cycle. This involves the use of a chemical indicator placed amongst the load or indicators incorporated in the sterilisation pouch. However these chemical indicators are not sufficient to ensure the autoclave cycles are running effectively. They are useful to distinguish which items have been sterilised from those to be done in so much as there is a change in the colour of the indicator during sterilisation. This change in colour will define those that have been through the autoclave cycle and those that have not. They must never be used and relied upon to replace the visual or printout log.

In large HSDU facilities, the autoclaves and washer/disinfectors are checked regularly and are taken out of service for these tests to be completed. There are also chemical indicators placed within the packs and loads to check effective sterilisation throughout the load. These tests are called 'Bowie-Dick' tests, and it is also possible to use these tests in vacuum phase autoclaves.

Autoclaves must be tested annually for insurance purposes, quarterly for safety checks, weekly for the door safety mechanisms, and daily for the cycle parameters.

It has long been known that handpieces present a specific problem where effective sterilisation is concerned. This is primarily due to the presence of internal lumen or water tubes which cannot be effectively sterilised in a displacement autoclave. They are more effectively sterilised in a vacuum phase autoclave when all the air is removed from the load during the vacuum phase of the cycle. Handpieces must be lubricated either before or after sterilisation, depending on the manufacturer's advice. To ensure effective lubrication, an oiling machine is advised to be used. This will deliver a measured amount of lubricant to the correct areas of the inside of the handpiece. If, in a dental practice, some are oiled before sterilisation and some after, then there must be separate machines or cans available both in the dirty area and the clean area. The same can or machine must not be moved from one area to another in order to prevent contamination of the clean area or items within it.

It is possible to purchase stand-alone handpiece lubrication and sterilisation units. They are relatively expensive and only sterilise small numbers of handpieces or their components, however the whole process can take as little as 8 minutes. It is certainly worthy of consideration for purchase in dental practices as they claim to effectively lubricate and sterilise handpieces.

For larger institutions using industrial sized facilities it is imperative that agreement is reached with the operators to ensure handpieces and their components are effectively lubricated and sterilised. Failure to do this at the contract negotiation stage could result in regular malfunction and considerable inconvenience to the user at a later date.

Storage and Use of Instruments

After the instruments have been sterilised and bagged, or sterilised in pouches, they must be stored correctly.

Instruments should be stored in dry conditions and used in rotation. They should not be stored where they can be damaged by steam or water and in such a way as to ensure the packaging is not ripped or damaged in any way. Any packet that is taken for use and found to be punctured or torn, must be discarded and the contents resterilised.

Trays of instruments processed in large facilities will be wrapped before sterilisation. The wraps used must be compatible with the autoclaves used and made of a material that is porous and allows steam to penetrate and sterilise the instruments inside. It must be strong enough to withstand ripping, tearing and puncture. This can be achieved by double wrapping. The outer wrap is designed to be a barrier to microbial penetration to allow the inner layer to maintain sterility, and is particularly important where packs are opened in an aseptic environment. When delivered to the hospital/clinic, they will be stored in a strict rotational order to ensure that the oldest is always used first. These items have a shelf life of one year.

Trays autoclaved and wrapped will have a processing date affixed with a 'use by' date. Items are usually 'sterile' for approximately a year after processing. There should be regular checks arranged to ensure that no item becomes 'out of date'. Should any item be found, then it has to be returned for reprocessing.

Items which are sterilised by other methods, i.e. gamma irradiated, will have a much longer shelf life, but checks should also be made to ensure items are used in rotation.

Transport of Instruments

Once the instruments have been sterilised they need to be moved to their place of use. In a dental practice, where local decontamination and sterilisation is carried out in situ, then the items will only have to be moved a short distance. In the case of a hospital, where decontamination and sterilisation is carried out in a large, off-site facility, then the items may have to be transported for some distance.

If moving from one room to another care should be taken not to drop the packets as this may cause damage to them. The instruments inside should be carefully wrapped in pouches to ensure sharp instruments do not puncture the pouches.

In larger institutions, where instruments are sent off-site, there must be rigorous arrangements to ensure compatible delivery and collection and to ensure instruments are available when needed. Details will need to be known of how the packs will be transported to ensure the integrity of the packaging. It is also imperative that the health and safety of the drivers and porters is not put at risk during the transfer of contaminated items. Contaminated items should be transported in locked trolleys that are specially designed to withstand a certain amount of impact damage. This is to ensure that there is little or no risk of exposure to the general public.

The pack should be checked when received at its intended destination and also when removed from its storage place. If any of these inspections reveal a break in the packaging, then the item must be reprocessed. Given the high cost in terms of both equipment and staff to effectively decontaminate and sterilise all medical devices, it would be wasteful in the extreme to then take scant regard of the processes employed when the sterile equipment is opened and used. Great care must be taken to preserve the sterility of the equipment and its surrounding environment when preparing it for use, and the techniques employed for this are known as 'aseptic techniques'.

Aseptic Techniques

Aseptic is defined as 'without micro-organisms'. An aseptic technique is carried out in a clean (as possible) environment using sterile equipment in a way that minimises the risk of transmission of infection.

An aseptic technique should be used whenever sterile or sterilised equipment is to be used. The whole purpose is to ensure the continued sterility of sterile items and the reduction of any risk of contamination before use. It is essential to use an effective aseptic technique when preparing for any surgical procedure. The whole area has to be kept as clean as possible and the instruments must not become contaminated.

It is equally important to ensure asepsis when preparing the surgery environment for non-surgical procedures. As previously stated instruments that cannot be packed when autoclaved cannot be considered sterile as they will have been contaminated by the environment on removal from the autoclave, but they will have been sterilised and that level of cleanliness must be maintained.

When preparing the surgery hand washing is important and appropriate changing of gloves between stages imperative. This has been outlined in a previous chapter. The instruments should remain in their pouches until required and only handled by gloved hands and then with as little contact with the working surfaces as possible. The nurse should be aware of not contaminating other unused packs and equipment not in packs and must develop techniques to ensure this continued asepsis.

When preparing an area for a surgical procedure the integrity of the sterile pack must not be compromised. It is essential that the operative field remains uncontaminated during the preparation procedure. To achieve this, certain physical barriers should be employed: sterile gloves, glasses, masks (with or without splashguard visor) and gowns which may be sterile or not and could be disposable. When laying up a surgical procedure, all the protective clothing should be put on before scrubbing up, i.e. the gown, mask and glasses and finally, after scrubbing up, the sterile gloves. It is important to ensure that the surfaces to be used to lay up the sterile equipment are clean and thoroughly disinfected before starting. A sterile cover should also be used to cover the surface. This is usually provided in a sterile pack which is unpeeled and put onto the decontaminated surface. When opening a sterile tray, the covers will act as a sterile cover.

Laying up a Parcel Fold surgical tray

If surgical procedures are carried out and no sterile gloves are available the nurse should not disregard the need for aseptic lay up techniques. They should perform scrupulous hand hygiene before putting on a clean pair of gloves. Do not be tempted to wash or alcohol-rub the gloves to 'make sure they are clean' as this reduces their efficiency — remember they are single use items and as such must never be washed or gelled.

Dental nurses should also wear some form of protective covering over their uniform. This should, ideally, be a gown but if not available then a plastic disposable apron is better than nothing. It is important to protect the uniform from blood contamination which is inevitable during a surgical procedure.

If no protective apron or gown is available, then the nurse's uniform will need to be washed separately from other washing and washed at a high temperature of at least 60°C to remove any blood-borne micro-organisms.

When ready to use the surgical tray the nurse should then lay out the surgical equipment on a clean cover after careful decontamination after the last patient and take every precaution to prevent accidental contamination of the clean area. A special fine bore surgical aspirator should also be available. These are available as disposable items and should be used as it is almost impossible to effectively decontaminate and sterilise the interior of a hollow instrument.

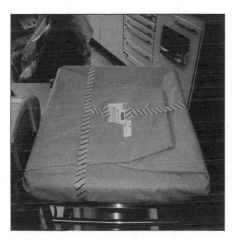

Figure 6. Unopened tray

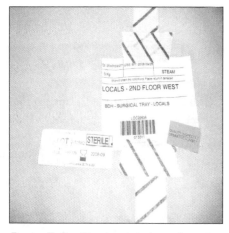

Figure 7. Sterilisation labels and tracing bar codes

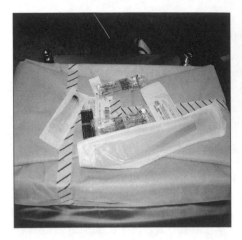
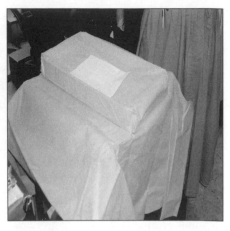

Figure 8. Disposable items ready to be opened

Figure 9. Outer layer opened, revealing inner second sterile cover

This cover can be opened before scrubbing up and putting on sterile gloves because there is the second sterile layer. The second layer must not be touched by unsterile gloves. It is possible to open the second sheet using one of the disposable items to be used during the procedure (*Figure 10*).

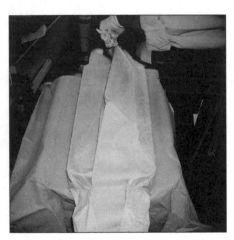
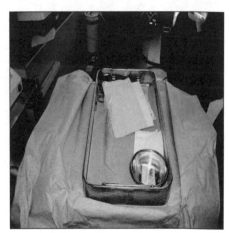

Figure 10. Opening layer before scrubbing up

Figure 11. Fully opened tray

These photographs show how a sterile disposable item can be partially uncovered and then, using the sterile part, used to draw back the sterile cover. In this case the disposable sucker tip is partially uncovered and then used to open the second layer. It is then fully uncovered and then dropped onto the sterile tray. Using this technique means that one nurse can lay up without having anyone else drop out the disposable items.

In *Figures 12* and *13* the nurse still has not scrubbed up or put on sterile gloves. *Figure 13* also shows how the disposable scalpel blade should be held in locked artery forceps and then applied to the Bard Parker handle. Alternatively a disposable complete scalpel can be used.

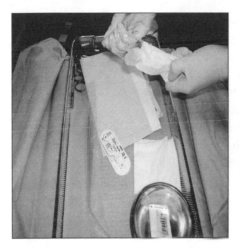

Figure 12. Dropping out disposable items before scrubbing up

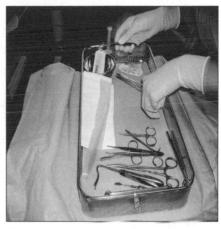

Figure 13. Putting blade onto scalpel handle using Spencer Wells artery forceps.

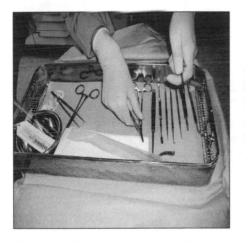

Figure 14. Putting instruments in order of use.

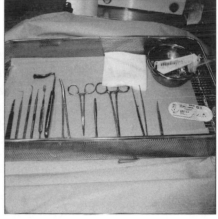

Figure 15. Complete lay up ready for use.

Instruments should be arranged in their likely order of use to minimise movement and handling of sterile instruments (*Figure 14*). The completed tray should be covered with another sterile sheet if it is not to be used immediately (*Figure 15*).

Specimens

If surgical procedures are being undertaken there is a reasonable chance that specimens will be taken of tissue removed (for example biopsy specimen) and there are very strict regulations about how these specimens are sent through the post.

It is important that the container holding the specimen is not contaminated with blood during the taking of the sample. The nurse and operator should be extremely careful not to touch the outside of the container with their contaminated gloves. The BDA (2003) gives detailed instructions as to how such specimens are handled. The packaging of the specimen, if unfixed, must comply with regulation UN 602 packaging requirements. This regulation ensures that certain strict tests have been carried out on the packaging, including drop and puncture tests. The package has to comply with strict packaging requirements and be clearly and conspicuously labelled on the outside. The outer packet must also be signed. If a dentist sends a specimen through the post without ensuring compliance with UN 602 they will be liable to prosecution.

If 'fixed' specimens are sent then they are not subject to such rigorous regulation but must still be carefully packed and conspicuously labelled as to the nature of the contents (for example *'pathological specimen – fragile handle with care'*). The outer cover must have the name and address of the sender or person to be contacted in the event of damage in transit. 'Fixed' specimens are those that have been killed and been preserved ready for examination.

Impression Materials and other Laboratory Items

It is the responsibility of the dentist to ensure that any items transferred to an external laboratory are decontaminated before sending and, where appropriate, a decontamination certificate is sent with the item to provide proof of effective decontamination.

The impression/appliance/denture must be thoroughly washed on removal from the mouth and continue to be washed until visibly clean. It should then be disinfected using a suitable recommended disinfectant. The item must be totally immersed in the disinfectant for the recommended time — spraying is not acceptable or effective. After immersion it should be washed again thoroughly and wrapped for transferral. If an alginate material is to be sent care must be taken to ensure that the impression is neither waterlogged nor allowed to dry out as either situation will lead to significant distortion of the impression.

Any products used to decontaminate and disinfect impressions, appliances or dentures must have the CE mark to demonstrate conformity to the European Directives. It is imperative to always follow the manufacturer's instructions for the dilution of the solutions and the soaking time needed for optimum disinfection.

Equipment to be sent for Maintenance or Repair

Equipment which requires maintenance or repair (for example handpieces) must be decontaminated and if suitable for sterilisation, sterilised before despatch to the outside technician. The equipment must have an appropriate decontamination certificate completed and sent with the item.

On return from repair or maintenance the item must be decontaminated, disinfected or sterilised before use.

Prions

The preceding information and advice about the cleaning, decontamination and sterilisation of medical devices is pertinent to all reusable, sterilisable medical devices. If carried out effectively and efficiently it will render the items micro-organism free and, therefore, safe to be used on the next patient. However there is one group of infectious agents that will not be destroyed by the processes outlined previously, however rigorously they are followed. That one exception is the eradication of prions.

Unlike other pathogenic micro-organisms, prions are not made up of cells and are not 'living'. They are mutant proteinaceous particles and as such are not destroyed by heat or steam under pressure. Instruments known to be infected by prions have to be dealt with in a completely different way.

There is a great deal of research being actively carried out into the way these particles form and their actions once inside the infected host. The most notorious disease in humans caused by prions is Creutzfeld-Jacob disease (CJD) and its variants (vCJD). These are diseases in a group called transmissible spongiform encephalopathies (TSEs). The disease has a devastating effect on those infected and is incurable. The incubation period for CJD or vCJD is anything from a few weeks to many decades.

Since its discovery and apparent spread, various committees and advisory groups have been set up to monitor the research and publish advice and guidance as necessary. One such body is the Engineering and Science Advisory Committee (ESAC) and also the Spongiform Encephalopathy Advisory Committee (SEAC). In its report SEAC (2007) recognised that there have been no cases of vCJD transmission arising from dental procedures reported to date. It concluded that:

'...preliminary research findings suggest that the potential risk of transmission of vCJD via dental procedures may be greater than previously anticipated. Although this research is incomplete...'.

SEAC, 2008

The report mentions the advice issued by the Chief Dental Officer in April 2007 (DH, 2007) and to conclude that to minimise risk it is critical that appropriate management and audit is in place, both for NHS and private dentistry. The report's final conclusion states that:

'The assessment will require continued updating as more evidence becomes available on the transmissibility of vCJD by dental routes, and on the prevalence of infection within the population...Given the potential for transmission via dentistry, consideration should be given to the urgent assessment of new decontamination technologies which, if proved robust and effective, could significantly reduce transmission risks'.

SEAC, 2007

A lengthy and comprehensive report issued by ESAC in 2006 looked in great depth at the problem of inactivating prions. It studied the work of Professor Robert Baxter et al (2006) at the University of Edinburgh. Professor Baxter and his team used high energy forms of gas, called plasmas, to strip contaminating molecules from instrument surfaces. Radio waves were used to excite the molecules of harmless gases. Once excited, the molecules and charged atoms (called ions and radicals) formed in the process effectively scour the surface of the instruments breaking down traces of biological tissue and convert them to non-toxic gases. This could prove to be a breakthrough in the search for affordable, practical ways of inactivating prions and effectively removing them from surgical instruments.

However, this process is still being developed and is not readily accessible, therefore other measures have to be taken to eliminate the risk of contamination being passed from one person to another via a contaminated instrument.

The current advice and agreed best practice is that as long as rigorous and effective standard precautions are followed and enforced then all instruments should be treated in the same way and be subjected to thorough cleaning, decontamination and sterilisation. It is widely agreed that certain types of tissue are more likely to harbour prions, these being:

- Brain tissue
- Neural or nerve tissue
- Lymphoid tissue
- Eye tissue.

Routine dental procedures will not involve contact with brain or eye tissue. Neural or nerve tissue will be involved in endodontic or root treatment of teeth when the pulpal or nerve tissue is removed to effect a root filling. Lymphoid tissue may be involved when biopsies are taken of lips or tongue or other intra oral tissues.

The Chief Dental Officer addressed the issue of root canal instruments in his letter in April 2007 when he said that all files and other endodontic instruments of a similar type must be single use only and must not be decontaminated and reused. This measure will help to reduce the small risk of prion contamination from pulpal tissue.

Instruments used to take biopsy specimens containing lymph tissue and the containers used to carry the specimen must be destroyed by incineration for patients with known or suspected vCJD. A technique should be used that prevents any contamination being transferred to the outside of specimen bottles. If disposable instruments are available their use should be carefully considered.

Instruments used when treating known CJD or vCJD-infected patients, must be rigorously decontaminated and sterilised. Again, if disposable alternatives are available they should be used (BDA, 2003).

References

Baxter RL et al (2006) Elimination of transmissible spongiform encephalopathy infectivity and decontamination of surgical instruments usingradio-frequency gas plasma treatment. *J Gen Virol* **86**(8): 76

BDA (2003) *Infection Control in Dentistry: Advice Sheet A12.* BDA, London

DH (2007) *Draft Health Technical Memorandum: Decontamination of Reusable Medical Devices.* Department of Health, London

DH (2007) *Important Advice for Dentists on Re-use of Endodontic Instruments and variant Creutzfeld-Jacob Disease (vCJD): Letter from Barry Cockroft, Chief Dental Officer for England.* DH, London

DH (2003) *A Guide to the Decontamination of reusable Surgical Instruments: NHS Estates.* DH, London

DH (2002) *Decontamination of Reusable Medical devices Standards.* DH, London

DH (2001) *Protocol for the Local decontamination of surgical Instruments: NHS Estates.* DH, London

DH (2001) *NHS Decontamination Project — Background and Expectations: NHS Estates.* DH, London

DH (1995) *Reporting of Injuries, Diseases and Dangerous Occurrence Regulations 1995*

(RIDDOR). HMSO, London

DH (1992) *Personal Protective Equipment at Work regulations 1992*. HMSO, London

ESAC (2006) T*he Decontamination of Surgical Instruments with Special Attention to the Removal of Proteins and Inactivation of any Contaminating Human Prions.* Engineering and Science Advisory Committee, London

Health and Safety Executive (1989) *The Pressure Systems and Transportable Gas Containers Regulations 1989*. Health and Safety Executive, London

Health and Safety Executive (2000) *Pressure Systems Safety Regulations 2000*. Health and Safety Executive, London

MHRA (2002) *Medical Devices Regulations*. Medicines and Healthcare Products Regulatory Agency, London

MHRA (1993) *Medical Devices Directive (93/42/EEC)*. Medicines and Healthcare Products Regulatory Agency, London

MHRA (1994) *Medical Devices Regulations (SI 1994 No 3017)*. MHRA, London

SEAC (2007) *vCJD and Dentistry — Position Statement*. Spongiform Encephalopathy Advisory Committee, London

CHECKLIST 5

Definitions:

- Cleaning
- Disinfection
- Decontamination
- Antisepsis
- Sanitisation
- Sterilisation

Legal requirements

The Decontamination Life Cycle

BDA Advice Sheet A12 Decontamination Flow Diagram

Decontamination Room / Area

- Dirty Area
- Clean Area

Decontamination Process

The Decontamination Life Cycle

- Cleaning / Disinfection
- Decontamination prior to sterilisation
  - Manual
  - Mechanical
    - Washer / Disinfectors
    - Ultrasonic Baths
- Wrapping
  - Pouches
  - Parcel Folds
  - Envelope Folds
- Sterilisation
  - Hot Air Sterilisation
  - Chemical Sterilisation

- Irradiation
- Steam Sterilisation
- Displacement Autoclaves
- Vacuum Phase Autoclaves

● Autoclave Care and Maintenance
● Storage and use of sterilised items
● Transport

Visible inspection at every stage

Aseptic Techniques

● Definition
● Process
● Procedure

Dealing with Specimens

Decontamination of Laboratory items

● Impressions
● Orthodontic appliances
● Dentures

Decontamination of items for maintenance or repair

Prions:

● Research
● Advice
● Current Practice

APPENDIX I

Legislation relating to the decontamination and sterilisation of medical devices.

Health Technical Memoranda (HTM)
HTM 2010 – Sterilisation.
HTM 2030 – Washer / Disinfectors.
HTM 2031 – Clean Steam.
(The 3 above will be superseded by HTM 01-01 when published in late 2007).
HTM 2025 – Ventilation in Healthcare Premises.

British Standards (BS)
BS 2646 – Laboratory Sterilisers.
BS EN ISO 13485 – 2003 – Guide to good manufacturing practicefor Medicinal Products – maintenance and validation.
BS 2745 – BSI – Washer / Disinfectors for medical purposes – Part1- Specification for General requirements.
BS – EN – 552 – Irradiation Sterilisation.
BS – EN – ISO 17665 – Moist Heat Sterilisation.
BS – EN – 556 – Sterile labelling.

Health Building Notes (HBN)
HBN 13 – Sterile Services Departments.

European Directives.
Directive 1995 / 1671 – Active Implantable Medical devices.
Directive 2000 / 1315 – In – Vitro Diagnostic Devices Directive.
Directive 2002 / 618 – Medical devices Directive.

Medical devices Agency (MDA), (now Medicines and Healthcare Products Regulatory agency MHRA) Directives
Device Bulletin DB 9501 – The reuse of Medical devices supplied for Single Use only.
Device Bulletin DB9605 – The purchase, Operation and Maintenance of benchtop Vacuum Steam Sterilisers.
Device Bulletin DB9804 – The Validation and Periodic testing of Benchtop Vacuum Steam Sterilisers.
HSG(93)26 – decontamination of Equipment prior to inspection, service and Repair.
(This list is not exhaustive, merely indicative).

CHAPTER 6

Safe Disposal of Clinical Waste, Sharps, Dental Instruments, Equipment and Materials

The disposal of waste of whatever type has been put at the top of the agenda since global warming has earned so much notoriety. Gone are the days when anything of no further use could be just thrown away without any thought of the consequences. It goes without saying that there are numerous Statutory Instruments and laws that govern the disposal of all and any items of waste. Failure to abide by these rules can result in prosecution, fines and even imprisonment, if found guilty.

Over the years, there have been many pieces of legislation covering the disposal of waste, including domestic waste and what can or cannot be flushed into the sewerage or drainage systems. In 2006, all this legislation was drawn together in one large document, the *Health Technical Memorandum (HTM) 07–01: Safe Management of Healthcare Waste* (DH, 2006). There is also extensive information and guidance in the British Dental Association (BDA, 2003). The main legislation which this document gives guidance and information for is the Hazardous Waste Regulations 2005 (DH, 2005).

The HTM guidance is not mandatory, but anyone not following the advice is advised to take alternative steps to comply with the legislation contained in the Hazardous Waste Regulations 2005.

The Health Technical Memorandum is published by the Department of Health but was compiled by a group of agencies, namely the Health and Safety Executive (HSE), the Department for the Environment, Food and Rural Affairs (DEFRA), the Department for Transport (DfT) and NHS Purchasing and Supply Agency (NHSPASA). This broad spectrum of expertise in the compilation of the document demonstrates how widely the implications of waste disposal spread. There are many Acts and regulations which have to be complied with in all aspects of the disposal of waste, the more important being appended for reference and guidance in *Appendix 1*.

It is imperative that local regulations concerning water and sewerage are followed, and the Environment Agency gives practical advice as Local

Authority regulations vary widely, some having much stricter recycling regulations than others.

HTM updates and revises guidance contained in the Hazardous Waste Regulations 2005 and takes into consideration legislation governing the management of waste, its storage, carriage, treatment and ultimate disposal and the health and safety requirements attached to these actions. It includes guidance on:

- Definition and classification of infectious waste
- Definition and classification of medicinal waste
- Changes in transport legislation
- Revised colour-coded, best practice waste segregation and packaging system
- The use of European Waste Catalogue Codes to identify waste
- Classification of microbiological cultures for carriage and disposal

This is written for all waste producers within the National Health Service and other healthcare providers and facilities.

The BDA (2003) gives clear advice on the segregation and treatment of clinical waste. It defines clinical waste as:

'Waste that is contaminated with blood, saliva or other body fluids and may prove hazardous to any person coming into contact with it.'

BDA, 2003

It is essential that each healthcare facility, however small or large, has robust policies and procedures in place for the safe segregation, disposal and transport of clinical waste. Large institutions, hospitals or personal dental service clinics will have policies in place, agreed at senior management level and which follow all the legislation. Waste management policies are often part of the control of infection policy and are given their own specific section.

Dental practices, whether NHS or private, should have a section dedicated to clinical waste management incorporated into their control of infection policies. The safe disposal of clinical waste is not confined to contaminated paper covers, used swabs or cotton rolls, used needles, etc. It also includes disposal of amalgam waste, spilled mercury, amalgam filled extracted teeth, waste developer and fixer, lead foil, etc. It is also important that instruments, equipment, materials and medicaments are discarded appropriately. None of these items can simply be 'thrown away'; they are either hazardous or chemical waste.

The BDA (2003) gives a categorical warning on the consequences of failure to comply with current legislation:

'A dentist who fails to dispose of waste in a safe manner will face prosecution by the authorities (Environmental Health Departments, Health and Safety Executive, etc) and may be liable to proceedings for serious professional misconduct before the General Dental Council (GDC). Clinical waste and hazardous waste must never be disposed of at local refuse tips or landfill sites.'

BDA, 2003

All Local Authorities have regulations in place and arrangements for the collection of such waste and they should be contacted for advice and that advice followed to the letter.

Dentists have an obligation to ensure that all and any staff who have to deal with clinical waste are adequately and appropriately trained and that the training is updated as necessary at regular intervals and in the light of changes in legislation. Training should be recorded and those records kept and made available for external audit, if requested.

Dental nurses should ensure they have up-to-date knowledge of local regulations and must be prepared to insist on appropriate training. Dentists have a duty of care under the Health and Safety at Work Act 1974 and are liable for the actions of their staff. By the same token, the staff have a duty of care to work in a safe manner and not put themselves or others in danger from their actions.

It is, therefore, essential that nurses are not only adequately and appropriately trained, but that they work in a safe manner and follow that training. It is also important that anyone else who may come into contact with the waste either before or after it is sealed, is adequately and appropriately trained in the safe handling of waste sacks, sharps bins, etc.

All staff that come into contact with or handle clinical waste must be protected by vaccination from hepatitis B and provided with appropriate personal protective clothing, as set out in the Personal Protective Equipment regulations. This should include disposable aprons, heavy duty rubber gloves and eye protection. They must also be trained in its use, when necessary.

Should any accidents occur when handling clinical waste, then they must be dealt with under the Reporting of Injuries, Diseases and Dangerous Occurrence Regulations (RIDDOR) and any inoculation injuries treated and reported appropriately. It is essential that anyone who handles waste when there is no-one else in the practice he or she knows what action to take in the event of sustaining an inoculation injury or other accident resulting from handling waste.

Laboratory staff must be aware of the need for careful disposal of any clinical or hazardous waste and particularly chemical waste.

There are environmental issues to be considered with the disposal of single use items. Many disposable items, aspirator tips, dappens pots, triple air syringe tips, etc. are disposed of in the clinical waste and sent for incineration. Endodontic instruments, burs and matrix bands are put into a sharps bin, again for incineration. Single use instruments are also disposed of in sharps bins and then incinerated. The residue from all this incineration is then often sent to landfill sites.

It is well documented that finding new sites is becoming increasingly difficult, and the environmental impact of using them and filling them with waste that will take hundreds of years to degrade is becoming unacceptable. If the number of disposable hand instruments used increases significantly there would be a detrimental impact on the environment despite the positive advantages of the reduction in the risk of cross-infection. Companies who make disposable hand instruments are actively seeking solutions to this dilemma. One suggestion is that the instruments are incinerated and that the residual metal is reused for non-medical uses. This would overcome any doubts that may exist about the indestructibility of prions and the continued prion contamination of the metal.

Each type of waste has its own procedure for safe handling and disposal. There are also strict regulations for the storage and transportation of the waste. Storage of large amounts of waste is a problem for larger institutions, but small dental practices must ensure that waste is stored safely until collected. There is also mandatory documentation required when the waste is moved.

Different Types of Waste

HTM describes the different types of waste and also describes the main responsibilities of each waste producer in line with the legal 'duty of care'. These responsibilities are:

- Describe the waste fully and accurately
- Complete and sign a waste transfer note (or consignment note for hazardous waste) prior to the waste being transferred to another party
- Pack waste securely (where appropriate) in line with the carriage regulations
- Store waste safely on site
- Register as a waste carrier (if required) and make all reasonable checks on waste carriers
- Select an appropriate recovery or disposal method
- Ensure waste falls within the terms of the waste contractor's Waste Management Licence, Permit or Exemption.

Amongst the legislation governing these requirements is:

- Waste Management Licences and Pollution Prevention and Control Permits
- Health and Safety legislation
- Consultation with Employees
- Transport legislation
- Procurement regulations
- EC Directive on Waste Electrical and Electronic equipment (WEEE).

There are many types of waste and many definitions of the differing types. HTM gives all these definitions but simplifies and unifies them into:

- Infectious clinical waste
- Hazardous/medicinal waste
- Offensive/hygiene waste
- Waste dangerous for carriage.

There are lengthy and complicated assessment processes to follow to identify which category the waste falls into. They can be simplified as follows:

- **Infectious Waste**
  - Waste that poses a known or potential risk of infection, regardless of the level of infection posed
  - Waste generated from healthcare practices or produced by community healthcare workers, is considered to be infectious waste unless a full assessment has taken place. This would be carried out by the healthcare worker on an item-by-item, patient-by-patient basis
  - Municipal or domestic waste is not considered to be infectious waste unless indicated by a healthcare worker, to be infectious. This also applies to waste from industrial sites.
  - Waste which contains non-infectious bodily fluids can cause offence and requires appropriate packaging. Such waste can be classified as offensive/hygiene waste.

- **Hazardous/medicinal waste**
  - Includes expired, unused, spilt and contaminated pharmaceutical products, drugs or vaccines that are no longer required and need to be disposed of appropriately

• Items contaminated from use in the handling of
pharmaceuticals, such as bottles or boxes, gloves, masks,
syringes and drug vials
• Hazardous waste includes:
>Amalgam
>Spent developer or fixer
>Amalgam filled extracted teeth
•Medicinal waste is divided into three groups:
>Cytotoxic and cytostatic
>Pharmaceutically active but not cytotoxic or
>cytostatic (in date drugs no longer required)
>Not pharmaceutically active and possessing no
>hazardous properties (out of date drugs
>for disposal)

Only cytotoxic and cytostatic medicines are classified as hazardous
waste, although some other medicines can possess hazardous properties.
Cytotoxic and cytostatic medicines are defined as possessing one or more
of the following properties:

• Toxic
• Carcinogenic
• Toxic for reproduction
• Mutagenic.

The Materials Data Sheets should be consulted as to whether any drug
or medicine has any of the above characteristics. It is extremely unlikely that
any dental practice would be concerned with any cytotoxic or cytostatic drug
or any other drug which may have those characteristics.

● **Offensive/Hygiene waste:**
• Is non-infectious and which does not require specialist
treatment or disposal but which may cause offence to those
dealing with it
• It does not need to be classified for transport
• It includes:
>Incontinence pads or other human hygiene waste
>Sanitary waste
>Nappies
>Medical/veterinary items or equipment which does
>not pose a risk of infection
>Animal faeces or soiled animal bedding.

Segregation of Waste

All waste produced needs to be segregated into appropriate containers of various colours. To make this segregation effective, staff must have:

- Background information and reasons for the segregation. This can take the form of posters, training materials and information leaflets
- Appropriate equipment, such as sufficient colour-coded waste receptacles. This includes colour-coded and labelled waste receptacles and sack holders, placed in safe positions but close to the production of the waste. Sack holders should be foot operated and have tight fitting lids. Receptacles must be replaced when no more than two-thirds full and securely closed when full and appropriately labelled. Collection should be at appropriate intervals for practices. Arrangements will need to be negotiated with the local authority or their registered licensed agents
- Clear and appropriate training and instruction.

The nationally recognised colour-coding is shown in *Figures 1* and *Figures 2* overleaf.

Colour	Description
	Waste which requires disposal by incineration Indicative treatment/disposal required is incineration in a suitably permitted or licensed facility.
	Waste which may be 'treated' Indicative treatment/disposal required is to be 'rendered safe' in a suitably permitted or licensed facility, usually alternative plants (ATPs). However this waste may also be disposed of by incineration.
	Cytotoxic or cytostatic waste Indicative treatment/disposal requires incineration in a suitably permitted or licensed facility.
	Offensive/hygienic waste* Indicative treatment/disposal required is landfill in a suitably permitted or licensed site. This waste should not be compacted in unlicensed/permitted facilities.
	Domestic (municipal) waste Minimum treatment/disposal required is landfill in a suitably permitted or licensed site. Recyclable components should be removed through segregation. Clear/opaque receptacles may also be used for domestic waste.
	Amalgam waste For recovery.

Note:
*The use of yellow/black for offensive/hygiene waste was chosen as these colours have historically
been universally used for the sanitary/offensive/hygiene waste stream.

Waste receptacle	Waste type	Example contents	Indicative treatment
'Over-stickers with the radioactive waste symbol may be used on yellow packaging	Healthcare waste contaminated with radioactive materials	Dressings, tubings, etc. from treatment involving low level radioactive isotopes	Appropriately licensed incineration facility
	Infectious waste contaminated with cytotoxic and/or cytostatic medicinal products	Dressings, tubings, etc. from cytotoxic and/or cytostatic treatment	Incineration
	Sharps contaminated with cytotoxic and/or cytostatic medicinal products	Sharps used to administer cytotoxic products	Incineration
	Infections and other waste requiring incineration including anatomical waste, diagnostic specimens, reagent or test vials and kits containing chemicals	Anatomical waste from theatres	Incineration
	Partially discharged sharps not contaminated with cytotoxic products	Syringe body with residual medicinal product	Incineration
Liquid Solid	Medicines in original packaging	Waste in original packaging with original closures	Incineration
Liquid Solid	Medicines NOT in original packaging	Waste tablets not in a foil pack or bottle	Hazardous waste incineration
	Infectious waste, potentially infectious waste and autoclaved laboratory material	Soiled dressings	Licensed/permitted treatment facility

(continued...)

Waste receptacle	Waste type	Example contents	Indicative treatment
	(1) Sharps contaminated with medicinal products[2] OR (11) Fully discharged sharps contaminated with medicinal products other than cytotoxic or cytostatic medicines	Sharps from phlebotomy	Suitably authorised incineration or alternative treatment facility[1]
	Offensive/hygiene waste	Human hygiene waste and non-infectious disposable, equipment, bedding and plaster casts	Deep landfill
	Domestic waste	General refuse[3] including confectionery products, flowers, etc,	Landfill
	Amalgam waste	Dental amalgam waste	Recovery

Notes:
1. The authorisation type and content for alternative treatments in Northern Ireland, Scotland, England and Wales may differ. Not all facilities are authorised to process the waste from (ii). It is therefore important that the waste description specifically indicates the presence or absence of the waste type identified in (ii).

Important: It is not acceptable practice to intentionally discharge syringes etc containing medicines in order to dispose of them in the 'fully discharged sharps receptacle. Partially discharged syringes contaminated with residual medicines should be disposed of in the yellow or purple lidded (if cytotoxic or cytostatic) sharps receptacle shown above.

2. The requirements for packaging are significantly affected by the presence of medicinal waste and the quantity of liquid present in the container.

3. General refuse is that waste remaining once recyclable items (for example paper and cardboard) have been removed.

Disposal of Waste

Radioactive waste: Has to be disposed of in suitably licensed facilities, normally by incineration.

Cytotoxic/cytostatic waste: Has to be disposed of by incineration in suitably licensed or permitted facilities. The waste is subject to the controls of the Hazardous Waste Regulations.

Infectious waste: Requires disposal by incineration in a suitably licensed and permitted facility. This includes anatomical waste and other types of waste which require incineration to comply with regulations. The waste is subject to the controls of the Hazardous Waste Regulations. This is waste contained in yellow sacks, bins, etc.

Sharps waste: Sharps are items that could cause cuts or puncture wounds or other percutaneous injury, including needles, syringes with needles attached, broken glass ampoules, scalpel and other blades and infusion sets. Orange lidded bins are for fully discharged sharps, if the syringe is partially discharged and contaminated, it should be disposed of in the yellow lidded bin. Sharps waste does not include:

- Bottles
- Vials
- Ampoules
- Tubes or tablets
- Swabs
- Other soft infectious waste.

Sharps waste should be incinerated in suitably licensed and permitted facilities.

Domestic waste: Waste similar to household waste and should not contain any infectious, infective or contaminated items. It is disposed of in black or clear bags.

Amalgam/mercury waste: The disposal of this waste is particularly pertinent to dentistry. It consists of amalgam waste in whatever form and includes any other materials contaminated with amalgam. It should be placed in rigid white containers which contain a mercury vapour suppressant. It must be sent to suitably licensed or permitted waste management facilities where the waste undergoes a mercury recovery process, prior to final disposal. Amalgam waste in whatever form must never be incinerated as this will release mercury vapour into the atmosphere. Mercury is a poison as is its vapour and prolonged exposure to mercury vapour will cause ill health and ultimately death.

Radiography fixer/developer: The treatment of this waste is of significance to dental healthcare facilities. Fixer/developer can be classified as hazardous waste depending on the type of materials used. Check with the manufacturer's material data sheet for precise details of disposal requirements. It should be sent, if appropriate, to a suitably licensed or permitted facility for material recovery. If recovery is not appropriate, fixer/developer should be incinerated at a suitable facility. It must never be washed down the sink into the sewerage system. If the waste is collected by licensed agents, then it must be stored safely in closed containers away from public access. The lead foil taken from radiograph packets prior to processing should not be put with other domestic or clinical waste. It must be kept separate for collection. It can sometimes be saved for charities who recoup money from companies who recover the lead from it.

Equipment: As far as is reasonably practicable, equipment should be decontaminated prior to disposal. Even after decontamination it may still have hazardous properties and is subject to waste management controls. If decontamination is impossible, then the waste contractor should be contacted to seek advice on treatment/disposal solutions. Disposal of large electronic equipment will need to be in accordance with the Waste Electric and Electronic Equipment Regulations (WEEE). Of particular concern to the dental profession is the disposal of mixing machines for amalgam as they could contain microscopic amounts of mercury, apart from the problems of decontaminating electric equipment used in the dental surgery.

Storage of Waste

Waste awaiting collection must be stored safely
For large facilities the storage area should be secure and covered and kept clear of loose bags. Dental practices must keep their waste for collection in a safe manner, out of the reach of the public or patients. Any area must be suitably labelled as a 'waste storage area' and kept locked at all times, except to allow addition of waste or collection. The area must be kept clean and no spilled waste allowed to stay there. It must also be kept free from vermin as far as is reasonably practical. This is to reduce the risk of bags becoming split open and the contents allowed to spill out. It must also be, as far as possible, weatherproof.

All staff should use personal protective equipment when handling the waste containers and receive training in safe handling. Staff should be monitored to check that they comply with the regulations agreed for the safe handling of the waste containers.

Before being taken to the storage area the various types of waste should be put into an appropriate receptacle. Waste receptacles of whichever type must not be filled more than two thirds full and then must be sealed. They must be securely sealed so that there is no chance of them being opened or of a bag opening after sealing. Sharps bins have an integral locking lid which locks into place and bags should be sealed using recommended closure ties. This is explained below.

Types of Waste Produced by Dental Surgeries

Contaminated waste: Paper covers, masks, swabs, disposable aspirator tips, etc. This should be put into yellow plastic bags and sealed when no more than two thirds full. The bags have to conform to EC regulations and are usually marked as clinical waste.

Domestic waste: Paper towels used for hand drying, packaging, office waste but not confidential waste. This waste should be put into black or clear plastic bags and again sealed when no more than two thirds full. They do not require any labels.

Sharps waste: Used for needles, endodontic irrigation syringes, discharged and partially discharged local anaesthetic cartridges, used burs, matrix bands and endodontic instruments, etc. Both hazardous and non-hazardous bins could be used, but not usually cytotoxic/cytostatic waste bins. The bins usually used will have either a yellow or orange lid depending on the waste contained, see above.

If any waste has been in the operating area of the surgery it should be considered as contaminated. It is for this reason that most dental surgeries will use only one sharps bin and usually a yellow-lidded bin. The bins must conform to British Standard (BS) 7320, United Nation packaging Group ii and EC regulations. Those made by reputable companies have the necessary labelling attached when bought, but usually have to be assembled. It is essential that they are assembled correctly and also closed correctly and the label completed with the date and name of the person assembling the bin and also the date and name of the person closing it. It must also have the place where it was used on the label.

The containers can have three different coloured lids, designating the different contents:

- Yellow body and orange lid: non-hazardous sharps
- Yellow body and yellow lid: hazardous sharps, which could include partially discharged local anaesthetic cartridges but not cytotoxic or cytostatic waste
- Yellow body and purple lid: cytotoxic and cytostatic waste only.

Amalgam waste: This includes waste amalgam, spent amalgam capsules, disposable containers used to hold the amalgam whilst being placed in the cavity, mixing machines, amalgam filled extracted teeth, and spilled mercury. If amalgam is mixed using the individual components, i.e. alloy and mercury, any receptacle or bottle which contained the materials or was used for mixing must be regarded as amalgam waste. All amalgam waste must be contained in a rigid white container which has a mercury suppressant in it. There should be separate containers for waste amalgam and spent capsules. Amalgam-filled extracted teeth should be washed and put into the waste amalgam pot, although amalgam recovery companies do now make a special receptacle for amalgam-filled extracted teeth. If disposable pots are used to hold the amalgam when being passed then they should be emptied of any residual amalgam and then they can be put into the yellow clinical waste bag. Even though amalgam must never be incinerated it is regarded as being very low risk for mercury vapour being emitted when these pots are incinerated in the waste. A sterilisable amalgam well should not be used as the amount of amalgam left will emit mercury vapour when autoclaved. If there is ever a mercury spillage then the mercury can be put into the waste amalgam container after clearing up using a suitable mercury spillage kit.

Confidential waste: Patient information, sensitive practice information, bank statements, receipts etc. should either be shredded and then disposed of in the domestic waste or sent for recycling, or placed in special 'confidential waste' bags which are then collected and disposed of by a licensed agent. If shredding in the practice it is advisable to have a cross-cut or confetti-cut shredder so that there is no chance of the documents being read.

Recyclable waste: Packaging, cardboard boxes etc. can be recycled as long as there is no possibility of them having been contaminated within the surgery environment.

Electrical equipment: Light machines, vitality testers, dental units, radiography machines, etc. must be decontaminated as far as possible before disposal. They cannot be disposed of at local authority waste centres as there is still a risk that they carry contamination. They must be disposed of by suitably licensed agents and have agreed decontamination documentation attached when collected. If an item cannot be decontaminated for whatever reason, then the waste disposal contractor must be contacted and arrangements made to ensure its safe removal and disposal.

Instruments: Used instruments that are broken or no longer required, should be decontaminated and, if possible, sterilised and disposed of using appropriate facilities. If, for whatever reason, they cannot be decontaminated they must be disposed of in a sharps bin. Instruments that still have a useful life but are no longer required should be decontaminated and sterilised and then they can be donated to dental charities that support under-developed and poorer countries (for example Dentaid). Single-use instruments should be placed in an appropriately sized sharps bin with either an orange or yellow lid. The bin should not be too large as it could create a manual handling risk because of its weight. It should also only be used for disposable instruments and designated as such on the outside.

Contaminated glass: Empty glass bottles and containers and pressurised canisters should not be put into incinerated waste containers. Pressurised canisters present an extreme risk to incinerator operators as they explode when heated, causing damage to the incinerator and its operator. Uncontaminated glass and canisters should be put into a special bin, similar to a sharps bin, but with an orange body and a black lid and usually of approximately 25 litres capacity. This container can also be used for broken glass. It should not be used for contaminated glass, whether contaminated by medicines or medicaments or by aerosol contamination, because it has been used close to the dental chair during treatment. Unbroken, contaminated glass can be wrapped securely in paper and then a plastic bag and placed in the yellow clinical waste bag. If the unbroken glass is securely wrapped and bagged then it will be contained if dropped and broken during the removal of the bag to its storage area. Broken contaminated glass should be put in a sharps bin.

Transport of Waste

The packaging of waste, its labelling and transport, are subject to rigorous control with documentation required at all stages to demonstrate compliance with legislation. This is designed to protect the transporter of the waste and the general public, who may come into contact with it should an accident occur during transit. Most large waste management companies have sealed specially constructed lorries to transport the packaged waste.

The waste is subject to the Carriage Regulations (see *Appendix 1*) which specifies the requirements for:

- Classification and identification: this is detailed in the European Waste Catalogue (EWC) and its codes. The EWC provides a common terminology for the designation of waste throughout Europe. It produces a long and complicated series of numbers and letters all of which lead to identification of the load contents, its point of origin and disposal requirements. This type of information is essential in the case of a load catching fire so that fire fighters are not put at risk. These codes need not be of concern to dental practices as they are more concerned with the vehicles containing the waste than the packaging of the waste, as long as the waste is packaged in accordance with the colour coded system above and labelled.

  •Packaging — This has been outlined previously
  •Marking — This has been outlined previously
  •Labelling — This has been outlined previously
  •Documentation — Agents and companies responsible for the collection and removal of waste will have documentation which must be completed prior to the waste being removed. The documents required include:

  Waste consignment note which provides information as to the number of packages and their type, name and address of consignor and consignee
  Waste transfer note which has to be signed by both the transferor (producer) and the transferee (recipient) both of whom keep a copy
  Consignment Notes which are available from the appropriate environmental regulatory agency. The use of such notes should be discussed with the company contracted to transfer the waste.

The BDA (2003) gives specific advice on the requirement for transfer notes; copies of transfer notes kept by the dentist will provide evidence of compliance with legislation if the practice is audited. Transfer and consignment notes must be kept for two or three years, depending on the waste transferred.

Packaging bought from reputable suppliers will most probably have the required information, i.e. 'clinical waste' labels, appropriate sharps bin labels, etc. already printed or fixed to the packaging, but the producer of the waste must ensure it is adequately and appropriately labelled and marked. They must also ensure that bags are securely fastened with approved ties.

It is important to reiterate that a dental practice must check with the local authority as to its current rules and regulations concerning the collection of clinical waste. Large facilities will need to negotiate contracts for their waste collection and disposal with suitably licensed and permitted agents and companies. It is the responsibility of the purchaser of the service to ensure that the licenses and permits are up-to-date and appropriate for the waste being contracted for removal. The managers responsible for negotiating the contract must ensure rigorous policies are in place to ensure that their responsibilities are met.

The management of clinical waste is a complex subject and could fill a book on its own to fully explore all its rules and regulations. This chapter has given background information and advice, particularly pertinent to dental practices. Larger institutions will have purpose-built and maintained areas for the safe storage of waste and will negotiate comprehensive contracts with recognised companies for the safe collection of the waste. They will have policies and procedures set up for the collection of waste from their clinical areas and surgeries and its transfer to the storage area, which will be rigorously enforced and regularly reviewed.

Dental practices do not generate large quantities of waste but need to ensure that procedures within their surgeries are the best possible to ensure safe transfer and collection. If there is any doubt as to the correct procedure to follow, the advice must be to check with the local authority or agency responsible for local waste collection. There is a large amount of advice available from the BDA and from Government agencies accessible on the Internet.

There is no doubt that non-compliance with local or national regulations will lead to serious consequences both from a legal point of view and from the General Dental Council.

References

BDA (2003) *Infection Control in Dentistry: Advice Sheet A12.* British Dental Association, London

DH (2006) *Health Technical Memorandum 07–01: Safe Disposal of Clinical Waste.* Department of Health, London

DH (1999) *Management of Health and Safety at Work Regulations 1999.* HMSO, London.

DH (1995) *Reporting of Injuries, Diseases and Dangerous Occurrences Regulations (RIDDOR) 1995.* HMSO, London

DH (1992) *Personal Protective Equipment at Work Regulations 1992.* HMSO, London

CHECKLIST 6

Legal Obligations

- HTM 07-01
- Hazardous Waste Regulations

Other Government Agencies

- Health and Safety Executive (HSE)
- Department of the Environment, Food and Rural Affairs (DEFRA)
- Department forTransport (DfT)
- National Health Service Purchasing and Supply Agency (NHSPASA)
- Types and definitions of Waste:
- Infections clinical waste
- Hazardous/medicinal waste
- Offensive/hygiene waste
- Waste dangerous for carriage.

Segregation of Waste

Colour Coding

Waste Packaging

Disposal of Waste:

- Radioactive waste
- Cytotoxic and cytostatic waste
- Infectious waste
- Sharps waste
- Domestic waste
- Amalgam/mercury waste
- Radiography fixer/developer waste

Storage of Waste:

- Types of waste produced in dental surgeries: Contaminated waste
- Domestic waste
- Sharps waste
- Amalgam waste
- Recyclable waste
- Electrical Equipment Waste
- Instruments
- Contaminated glass
- Transport of Waste
- European waste catalogue

APPENDIX I

Legislation relaying to clinical waste management:

- The Carriage of Dangerous Goods and use of transportable Pressure Equipment regulations 2004
- The Controlled waste Regulations 1992
- The Controlled Waste (Registration of carriers and Seizure of Vehicles) regulations 1991
- The Control of Substances Hazardous to Health Regulations (COSHH) 2002
- Environmental Protection (Duty of Care) Regulations 1991
- The Environmental Protection Act 1990
- The Hazardous Waste (England and Wales) Regulations 2005
- The Health and Safety at Work Act 1974
- The Health and Safety (Consultation with Employees) Regulations 1996
- The Ionising Radiation Regulations 1999
- The Landfill (England and Wales) Regulations 2002
- The Lists of Wastes (England) Regulations 2005
- The Management of Health and Safety at Work Regulations 1999
- The Medical Devices Regulations 2002
- The Misuse of Drugs Regulations 2001
- The Personal Protective Equipment at Work Regulations 1992
- The Pollution Prevention and Control (England and Wales) Regulations 2000
- The Public Contracts Regulations 2006
- The Radioactive Material (Road Transport) Regulations 2002
- Radioactive Substances Act 1993
- The Reporting of Injuries, Diseases and Dangerous Occurrences Regulations 1995
- The Waste Incineration (England and Wales) Regulations 2002
- The Waste Management Licensing Regulations 1994

European Legislation:

- Council Directive 75/442/EEC 1975
- Council Directive 01/689/EEC 1991
- Council Directive 1999/31//EC 1999
- Council Directive 2002/96/EC 2003

Numerous and various advice from Government agencies including:

- Department of Health
- Health and Safety Executive
- Department for Transport
- Environment Agency — Guidance Leaflet WM2

This list is by no means exhaustive, merely indicative.

Index